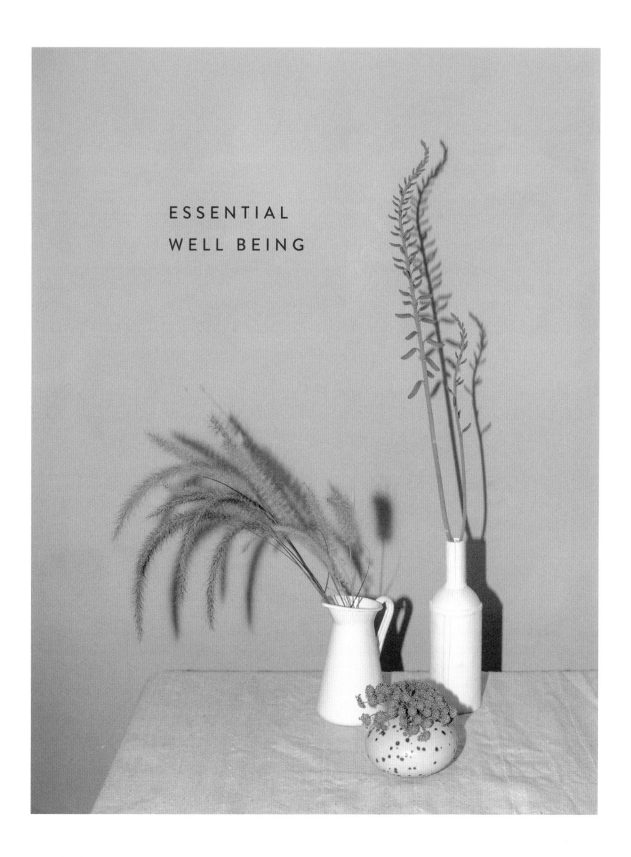

ESSENTIAL
WELL BEING

ESSENTIAL WELL BEING

A Modern Guide to Using Essential Oils

in Beauty, Body, and Home Rituals

SARA PANTON

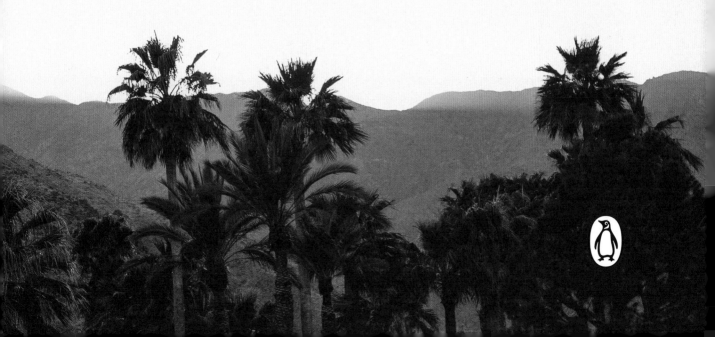

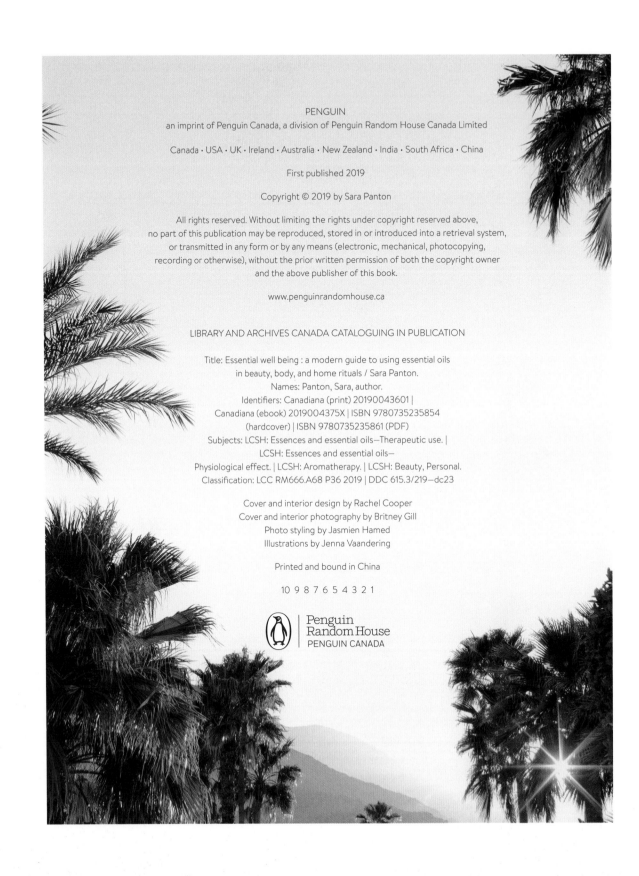

PENGUIN

an imprint of Penguin Canada, a division of Penguin Random House Canada Limited

Canada · USA · UK · Ireland · Australia · New Zealand · India · South Africa · China

First published 2019

www.penguinrandomhouse.ca

LIBRARY AND ARCHIVES CANADA CATALOGUING IN PUBLICATION

Title: Essential well being : a modern guide to using essential oils
in beauty, body, and home rituals / Sara Panton.
Names: Panton, Sara, author.
Identifiers: Canadiana (print) 20190043601 |
Canadiana (ebook) 2019004375X | ISBN 9780735235854
(hardcover) | ISBN 9780735235861 (PDF)
Subjects: LCSH: Essences and essential oils—Therapeutic use. |
LCSH: Essences and essential oils—
Physiological effect. | LCSH: Aromatherapy. | LCSH: Beauty, Personal.
Classification: LCC RM666.A68 P36 2019 | DDC 615.3/219—dc23

Cover and interior design by Rachel Cooper
Cover and interior photography by Britney Gill
Photo styling by Jasmien Hamed
Illustrations by Jenna Vaandering

Printed and bound in China

10 9 8 7 6 5 4 3 2 1

Penguin
Random House
PENGUIN CANADA

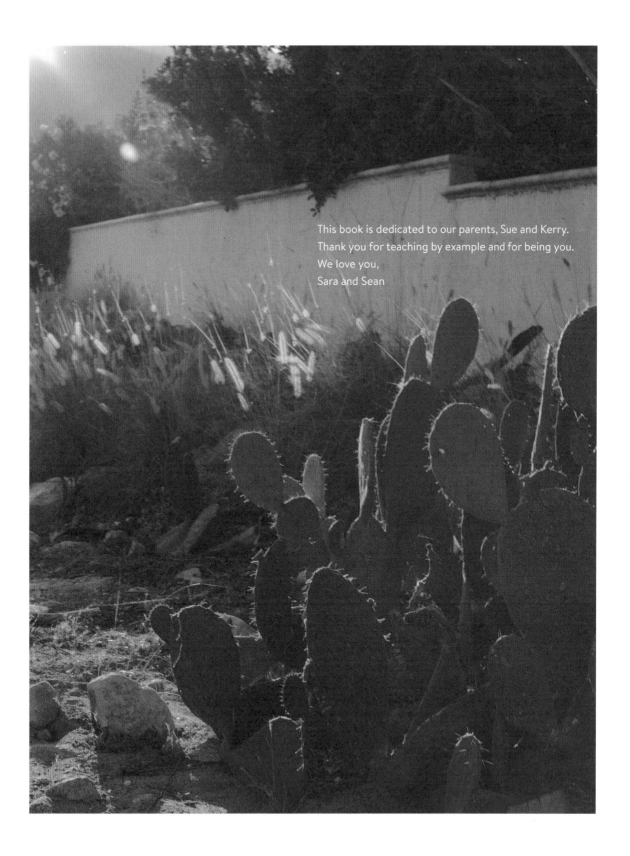

This book is dedicated to our parents, Sue and Kerry.
Thank you for teaching by example and for being you.
We love you,
Sara and Sean

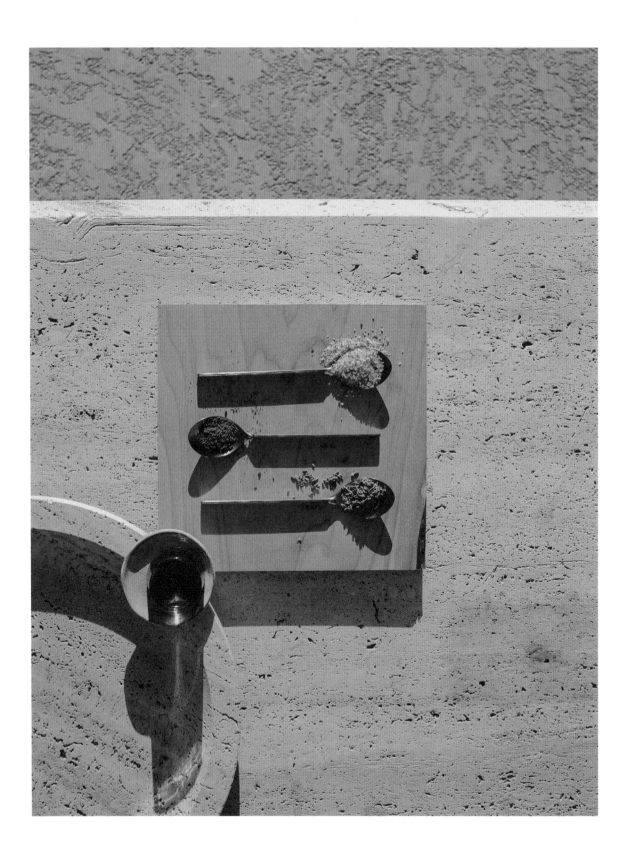

CONTENTS

BEAUTY

MORNING BEAUTY RITUALS

AFTERNOON BEAUTY RITUALS

EVENING BEAUTY RITUALS

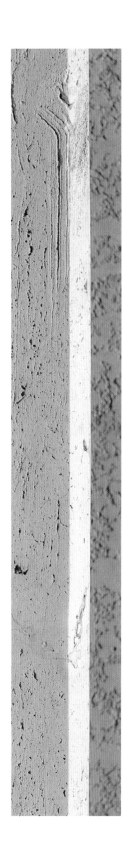

BODY

MORNING BODY RITUALS

AFTERNOON BODY RITUALS

EVENING BODY RITUALS

HOME

KITCHEN

BATHROOM

LIVING ROOM

BEDROOM

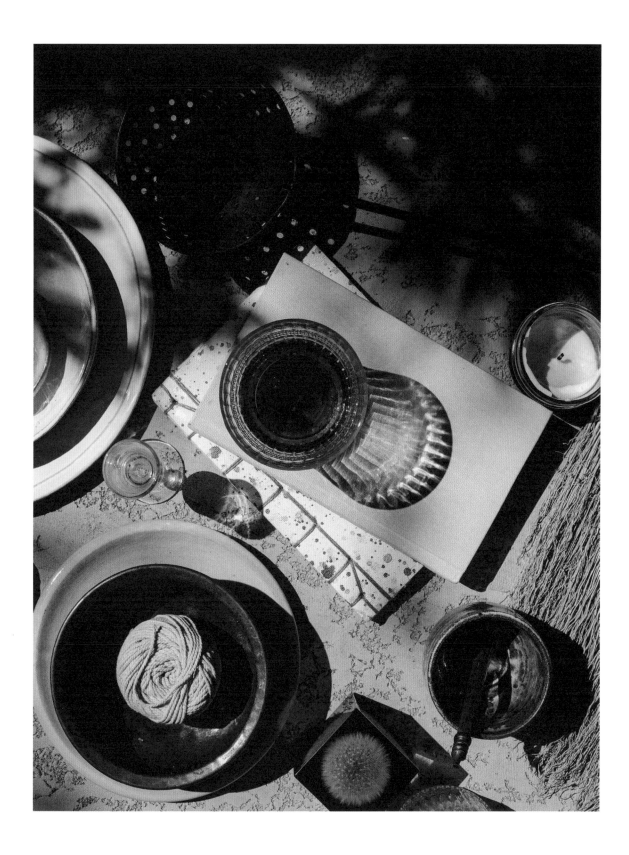

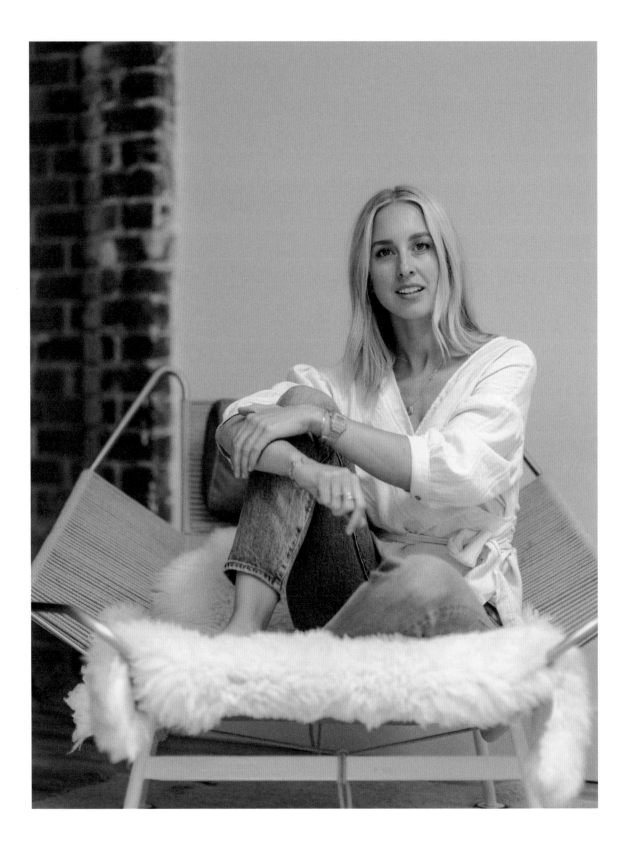

INTRODUCTION

My life over the past few years has been dynamic, to say the least. Building a company from a passion project comes with a lot of risks and many moments spent in the discomfort of the unknown. Despite years of late nights followed by early mornings and many lessons of patience and diligence, I wouldn't have it any other way.

Living in the relentless momentum of entrepreneurship has forced me to think creatively about the ways I fit personal wellness into my day. After building vitruvi, a wellness company, and seeing all the different ways it can be approached, I believe that the pursuit of living naturally and finding "balance" can get overly complicated pretty quickly. My approach and the philosophy of vitruvi is quite the opposite. I believe that we can create and carve out simple (even secret) moments throughout our days to reconnect with ourselves, find perspective and restore our energy.

In this book, you'll find more than 100 DIY essential oil recipes, small rituals, tips and suggestions that create what I believe to be a well-rounded experience for living. This isn't a complex 10-day plan or 21-day detox for living more naturally—this book is composed of recipes that you can pick and choose from depending on how you are feeling and what your body (and home) need at a particular time, daily habits and beautifully simple botanical practices from around the world that I have collected over the years, either through my own experimentation while working on my degree in global health or by interviewing people I admire. For example, you'll find a leg stretch to try while doing a simple face steam, or an ancient pressure point technique to try on your hand after you use a focusing mist at your work desk. The essential oil recipes all take less than 15 minutes of your time to create and are organized into three sections: Beauty, Body and Home. Each section is further organized by moments of your day or rooms of your house. It's meant to guide you through specific rituals for morning, afternoon and evening and to help you incorporate botanical-based products into more rooms of your home. My suggestion for how to use this book is to first sit quietly and think about what daily rituals or spaces of your living environment you would like to be more natural, then go from there.

For centuries, moments of self-care have been times to reconnect with yourself, and the intention of this book is to get back to this—it's not about wellness for the sake of wellness but about creating moments that leave you with a little more inspiration and energy to take on whatever work or pursuit you believe is important. Each day, as I make my morning matcha and get ready to go to the office, I revisit my intention: creating products and content for women that inspire them to nurture and take care of themselves, so that they will have a little more energy, stamina and inspiration to go into the world each day and make a positive impact. If these little bottles and simple recipes offer even a sliver of what I envision for you, I will be so very happy.

Take care,
Sara

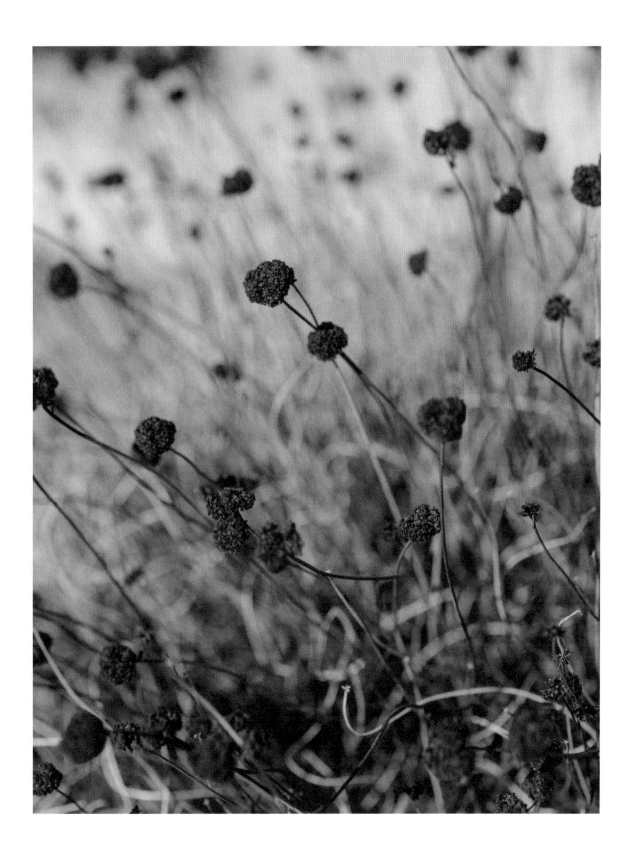

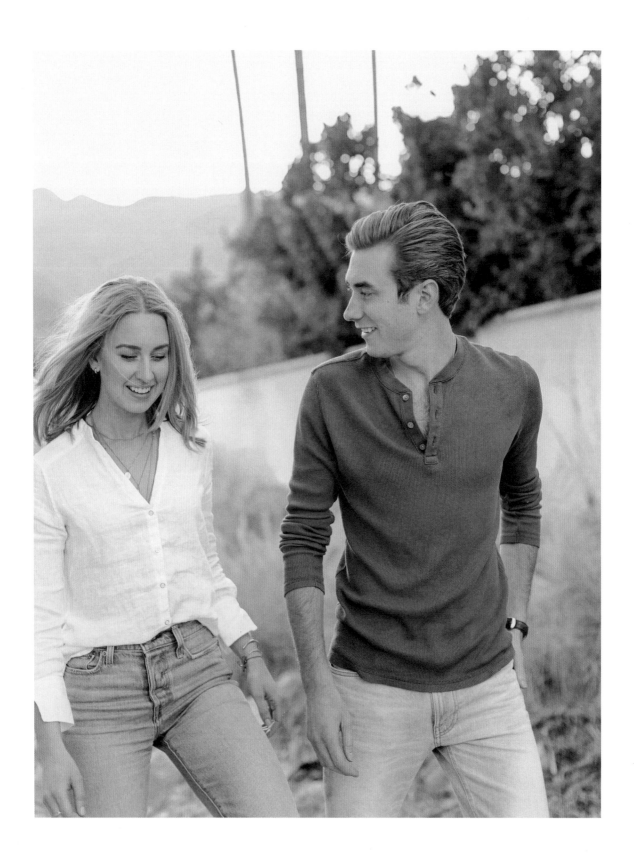

OUR STORY

We grew up in a small farming community on an island off the west coast of Canada. This idyllic place was a mixture of farms and ocean. Growing up on the beach, my brother Sean and I were two of the few kids in the area, so becoming friends was basically a necessity—play together or alone. We would spend our evenings and weekends building beach forts, collecting berries from farm stands and paddle boarding. Although at the time we didn't fully understand the beautiful simplicity we lived in, we now appreciate how our parents were early adopters of organic produce, non-toxic cleaning products and an overall curiosity about health and well-being.

Needless to say, our belief in natural and simple living came from our mom and dad. They were very influential in the way we regard nature and our respect for the natural world. As a family, we would frequently go hiking or camping and spend time outdoors, planting our own vegetables and picking apples with our grandparents. We didn't travel internationally during our childhood, nor were we introduced to business, yet I was always curious about cultures and places around the world, and Sean was always very entrepreneurial.

I knew I was interested in wellness and wanted to help people, so I decided pretty early on that I wanted to be a doctor. I felt that a career in medicine would allow me to travel, and I knew that I wanted to practise medicine for people who wouldn't otherwise have access to it. I began working on a degree in Global Health Sciences, and throughout my studies, my grandfather (Papa) would often remind me "to think smart, not hard" and to "keep my options open." I'm very glad I did, because it made me stay curious about the themes, subjects and topics that light me up.

In university, I made my first trip abroad with my dad. We took out an old-world atlas and chose a spot on the map: Morocco and Spain. In Spain, I came to love Mediterranean culture, fresh food, coffee, olive oils and tapas. Morocco was fully immersive—we took a train through the entire country, stopping at small towns, walking through souks, collecting herbs, drinking the iconic sugar-filled peppermint tea in the morning and discovering hidden fabric and leather dyeing operations. The most transformative experience of Morocco for me was witnessing the way spa culture is fully integrated into their way of life. It was not a frivolous, once-or-twice-a-year experience—as it is for women in North America. Instead, the hammam was ingrained in their everyday and weekly routines. Dry brushing, steam rooms, exfoliation, black soap and rose-infused body oils were all an unwritten part of life. I loved learning about the ways that people would take care of their skin and create rituals that helped their bodies and minds reset. On this trip, I started to collect dried rose petals, peppermint tea, frankincense and black soap, which sparked a new love for self-care in me, as well as a curiosity about how I could use ancient rituals to elevate the simple moments of my day.

Another travel experience that dramatically influenced my passion and inspiration for what has become vitruvi was my first trip to Kenya. I spent time in Masai Mara working with women's cooperatives as a member of the Nobel Prize–nominated charity WE.org. I worked with the organization for 5 years: from the time I left high school until I completed my university degree. At that time, the now-massive organization was very grassroots, and the entire team flew to Kenya to witness firsthand the positive impact we were creating in partnerships with the communities there. I walked with women to collect water from the Mara River, talking to them about their husbands, their children and how empowerment through alternative income projects enabled them to take care of themselves and their families. These conversations were transformative but not in the way that you might expect—they instilled in me a deep desire to devote my life to helping women take care of themselves. In my mind, there is nothing more powerful than a woman who is self-sufficient: a woman who is strong in her body and in her mind and who knows how to tend to her overall wellness. That is a powerful woman.

After receiving my degree in Global Health Sciences, I had to transition from studying health from an anthropological perspective to the scientific rigour of medical school. It was a big change, but it provided me with a deeper understanding of physiology, the endocrine system and body systems. A certain alchemy happened for me while studying medicine—I became passionate about learning about rituals and how people could reconstruct their days and habits to better address their potential. The concept of personal potential, self-care and botanicals became my passion, and that passion translated into an outlet that was a website.

My brother and I never set out to build a company. We were roommates—Sean studying entrepreneurship and myself in medical school. We started a simple website that Sean would work on in the evenings, while I interviewed people in our community and people I met in school about their health and wellness practices. We started experimenting with essential oils after referencing the products, ingredients and botanicals I was writing about from cultures around the world. We kept things simple at the start by creating our own blends to help us study, to wake up in the morning and to fall asleep in the evenings. These first blends are the foundation of our Rituals Collection product line.

We became passionate about learning how scent specifically could help cue the brain and body to transition through moments of the day. Our first collections were built in our apartment—we were filling bottles by hand, finding creative ways to blend oils, learning about their benefits and experimenting on friends and family. We offered a simple initial collection on our website that's still very much the basis of what the company has expanded into today.

The desire and pursuit that inspired me to want to be a doctor are the same ones that inspire and fulfill me every day at our office. To travel, to act as a translator between cultures and practices and to help people carve out moments for themselves throughout their day—that's what drives me. Our products, content and ethos are meant to act as small reminders that you can transform the simple moments of your day into moments when you fill your cup back up. Moments when you explore your own potential through the simple and ancient act of taking time for your body and mind using botanicals, plant oils and rituals.

We launched the concept for vitruvi and our initial collection (which had paper labels . . . not the best idea when creating an oil product) and quickly started gaining traction. We started by taking orders from boutiques in Canada and then expanded that to include North America. For the first 2 years of the company, we hand-filled and hand-parcelled every single order. This attention to detail and direct relationship with our customers and stores built the foundation of the company to be completely customer-centric. By asking for feedback, creating iterations and sourcing and cultivating larger volumes of products, Sean built the entire operations of the company without any experience at the age of 22. We were learning on the fly: our days were spent talking to customers and boutique wholesale accounts and our evenings were spent mixing oils, filling bottles and preparing shipments. The wellness industry was just starting to gain traction, and with that, the company did as well.

What has resulted is so much more than we could have ever imagined. Our customers are some of the kindest and most inspiring people we have ever met. Our story is something that is still being written every day. As brother and sister, we come into the office each morning to a team of talented, compassionate, intuitive and creative people who feel like family. vitruvi is built out of passion and the happy coincidences that can happen only when you are in flow—when you take risks and follow a path that feels uncomfortable but also very true to you and what you want to contribute to the world. We feel lucky every day to be able to experiment, design, cultivate, create and produce products that embody what we hope for our customers.

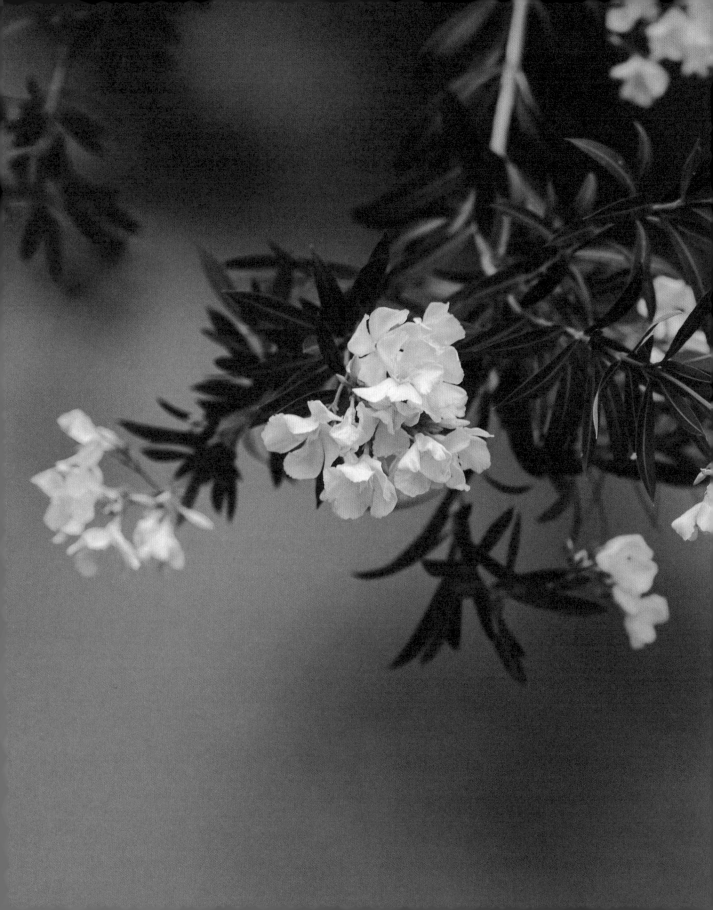

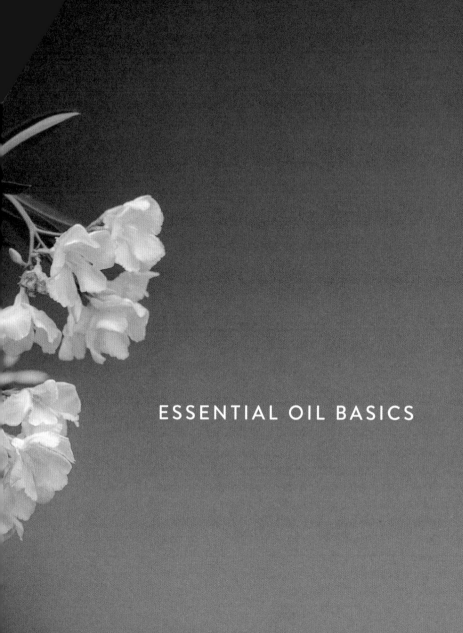

ESSENTIAL OIL BASICS

Before you dive in, I want to share some information that I think will be helpful in understanding what essential oils are and where they come from. This section can help guide you when you're purchasing essential oils, and it also provides context for all the recipes you'll find in this book. If you're new to experimenting with essential oils and plant-derived oils, hopefully this section gives you a solid foundation to start with and answers some of the questions you may have.

WHAT ARE ESSENTIAL OILS?

Essential oils are extracts from flowers, leaves, barks and resins. They are the components of plants that contain the chemical molecules that give the plants their intrinsic aromas. On a superficial level, they smell amazing and are a completely natural way to scent your living spaces (as well as yourself) without chemicals and synthetic fragrances. Beyond their superficial benefits, essential oils also contain some of the most concentrated and potent extracts of a plant. This intense concentration means that different oils contain properties that are antimicrobial, antibacterial, antiseptic, astringent and even anti-inflammatory.

All plants contain essential oils—they are volatile chemical compounds that are necessary for the plant to survive and are found in greater or lesser quantities depending on the plant, botanical or fruit. Essential oils are different from plant-derived oils in that they don't have any nutritional value and evaporate into the air. They also offer little moisture benefit to the skin, unlike coconut and avocado oils, which contain natural fats and omega fatty acids that make them moisturizing for the body topically as well as internally. The degree to which certain plants make volatile chemical compounds known as "essential oils" makes these oils more or less available to produce on a larger scale. Some botanicals make so little that it cannot be extracted, whereas others (such as sweet oranges and lavender) make enough that it is cost effective and easy to extract. The availability, ease of extraction and stability make some essential oils more or less expensive than others.

HOW ARE ESSENTIAL OILS MADE?

There are two main methods we use to extract essential oils. The first is steam distillation, which is also the way aromas for perfumes were historically made in France. In this extraction process, steam is passed through the plant materials, whether that be bark, flower petals or herbs. The heat and gentle pressure from the distillation apparatus interact with the oils in the plants, and they evaporate into the steam. These tiny droplets of steam-suspended essential oils are then concentrated and collected through a cooling condenser that turns the steam into water and separates the essential oils from the water as it cools. The two products that result are pure essential oil and hydrosol (infused water). The hydrosol makes a beautiful natural toner.

The other method for extracting oils is cold pressing. Cold pressing is used to extract oils mainly from citrus peels and rinds, but it can also be used with other fruits and vegetables, such as avocados. Much as you would create a high-quality olive oil, cold pressing involves the simple practice of crushing rinds and peels from fruits such as grapefruits, lemons and oranges.

WHAT SHOULD I LOOK FOR WHEN BUYING ESSENTIAL OILS?

The main thing to consider, above all else, is whether you're purchasing oils that are 100 percent pure. This means there are no synthetics, fillers, contaminants or diluters mixed in with the oil. If you've been reading up on essential oils already, you may have come across the term *therapeutic grade*. This isn't actually an industry standard—it's a trademark that certain essential oil companies use to regulate their products. So, oils can still be 100 percent pure, ethically sourced and even organic without having this label on them. Your best bet is to do a little research and find out directly from the company what its stance is on sourcing and quality. Another thing to look for is matte packaging—oils packaged in matte bottles allow less oxygen and light to reach the oils, which can alter the stability of oils that are photosensitive, such as citrus oils. The bottom line: look for oils that are protected from light and oxygen with a dark bottle and dropper lid and for oils that are certified organic when possible and always 100 percent pure.

ESSENTIAL TOOLS FOR BLENDING AND ENJOYING ESSENTIAL OILS

Building a small collection of tools for the products you're going to make may seem like adding more "stuff" to your home, but these tools will become household items that you'll use over and over again. For this reason, I tend to lean toward more sustainable materials, like glass, when it comes to containers or bottles—that way I can reuse an item multiple times and don't have to worry about any plastic interacting with the essential oils. If you are going to use plastic, just make sure to follow the storage instructions correctly, especially if they mention to keep it in a cool, dry place away from direct sunlight. These suggestions are simply a guideline, and they reference tools I've developed a preference for during my experimentation. I hope you enjoy setting up your own tool kit or shelf in your home and that you'll take the time to invest in a few simple accessories that inspire you to build natural, simple and clean products.

DROPPER BOTTLES

Most of the dropper bottles you can find will be made of either clear or dark amber glass. Depending on the length of time that you are hoping to store a product, dark glass helps protect the oils from UV rays, which can damage the oils and make them less effective, as well as decrease their aroma. More importantly, some essential oils can undergo a chemical change that makes them more sensitive for the skin if exposed to too much light. A great rule of thumb is to think about how you will be using the product you are making and where you will be storing it. If you can't ensure that it will be out of direct sunlight most of the time (especially for photosensitive citrus essential oils), then I would suggest using a dark glass dropper bottle whenever possible. Otherwise, clear glass dropper bottles are a great option, especially because you can tell how much product you still have remaining.

SPRAY BOTTLES

Spray bottles are great to have for different rooms of the house, especially for recipes such as linen and shower sprays. I love making sure that the handle of the bottle is comfortable for misting around your home and that the spray is fine enough that the liquid you are spraying distributes evenly. You can find spray bottles in a variety of materials, but I prefer using a clear glass bottle so I can see how much product I have left. You're welcome to use a dark glass bottle as well if you're worried your product will be exposed to some sunlight.

MIST BOTTLES

Mist bottles are smaller than spray bottles and offer a more fine distribution of liquid for uses such as face mists and hair perfumes. Using a smaller volume makes it easier to fit in your hand as well as to take on your travels. Again, a glass bottle (dark or clear) is preferable, but you can also use plastic if you're concerned about travelling with glass.

JARS

I love using dark glass jars for scrubs and deodorizing recipes. The most important thing to look for when buying glass jars, especially ones that you'll use for shower scrubs, is to ensure that they have a tight seal for keeping water out, as this will help to extend the product's shelf life.

ALUMINUM TINS

These are great for making balms and salves because the aluminum material helps keep the temperature of the semi-solids consistent. Tins are also super easy to throw into your bag, and most of them come with a twist lid that will ensure you don't end up with an open balm in your purse.

DIFFUSER

For diffusing essential oils in your space, we love using an ultrasonic diffuser. This means it distributes essential oils evenly into the air by oscillating small movements on a plate without any heat, so the diffuser itself runs through vibrations. Because of this, the plastic inside the diffuser, the water you pour into it and the oils are never heated, which means the plastic has no interaction with the essential oils. We also recommend choosing a diffuser that uses BPA-free plastic. Looking for a diffuser with a safety-off switch is a good choice, so you can set it and forget it.

TOWELS

For cleansing your face as well as for covering your head while doing face steams, having a set of favourite bathroom and kitchen towels can elevate any moment. As with any material we put on our body, I love using an organic cotton or linen fabric, which ensures both that the texture of the material is natural and that the fabric hasn't been processed with synthetic detergents or artificial dyes. Natural fibres sometimes have a slightly rougher feel to them, but this texture can offer a slightly exfoliating treatment when patting dry the skin on the face or drying off after a shower.

FACE PADS

Instead of using disposable cotton pads, I try to use reusable pads made of natural cotton fabric. I just cut up the fabric into smaller pieces and then reuse them for taking off makeup, wiping my face clean of face masks or applying natural toners. Reusable face pads are easier on both the environment and your skin.

BOWLS

When mixing and creating products, I love using a ceramic bowl because the weight helps keep the bowl on a surface if I am whisking or mixing briskly. The natural material of the clay also helps keep the temperature of the product you're creating consistent. I find that using a glass or metal bowl can often transfer heat from my hands or the ingredients through the material, which is another reason I love ceramic bowls. Avoid using plastic bowls for mixing anything, especially essential oils, because plastic is an unnatural substance and the essential oils can affect its integrity, making it less stable.

DRY BRUSH

When choosing a dry brush, always select a natural bristle brush that is organic and made with a long, sustainable bamboo handle, if possible. I love using a brush with a long handle because it allows easy brushing of the back as well as the back of the legs and thighs. When storing your dry brush, make sure to keep it out of moisture. Also, clean it regularly with tea tree and water to ensure that bacteria from your exfoliating doesn't build up in the brush.

GLOSSARY OF ESSENTIAL OILS

There are hundreds of essential oils available throughout the world. I've decided to highlight a few of the most versatile ones that can be used throughout your life in a range of ways. These are the essential oils I'll reference and refer to throughout the book. Here is a summary of why I chose them and a few quick tips on how they can be used and blended.

FLORAL

Geranium
PROPERTIES: balancing, sensual
GREAT FOR: beauty, skincare, bath
WHY I LOVE IT: it's the ultimate feminine aroma
BLENDS WELL WITH: frankincense, eucalyptus, peppermint

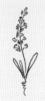

Lavender
PROPERTIES: antibacterial, anti-inflammatory, soothing
GREAT FOR: bedtime, bath, skincare, travel
WHY I LOVE IT: it smells like France in a bottle
BLENDS WELL WITH: eucalyptus, ylang ylang, cedarwood

Ylang ylang
PROPERTIES: calming, nourishing
GREAT FOR: bedtime, bath, beauty, skincare
WHY I LOVE IT: it smells and feels super luxurious
BLENDS WELL WITH: lavender, geranium, lemon

CITRUS

Bergamot

PROPERTIES: comforting, cleansing
GREAT FOR: skincare, bath, stress
WHY I LOVE IT: it reminds me of a warm cup of Earl Grey tea
BLENDS WELL WITH: grapefruit, geranium, cedarwood

Grapefruit

PROPERTIES: brightening, energizing
GREAT FOR: skincare, cleaning
WHY I LOVE IT: it's fresh and light without being too sweet
BLENDS WELL WITH: bergamot, sweet orange, spruce

Lemon

PROPERTIES: antibacterial, uplifting
GREAT FOR: cleaning, laundry, mood
WHY I LOVE IT: it freshens up every room in the house
BLENDS WELL WITH: bergamot, frankincense, spruce

Sweet orange

PROPERTIES: brightening, astringent
GREAT FOR: skincare, cleaning, bath
WHY I LOVE IT: it smells like a fresh glass of orange juice
BLENDS WELL WITH: peppermint, rosemary, eucalyptus

HERBAL

Eucalyptus

PROPERTIES: antibacterial, invigorating

GREAT FOR: shower, travel, stress

WHY I LOVE IT: it brings the feeling of a spa to wherever you are

BLENDS WELL WITH: cedarwood, lavender, sweet orange

Lemongrass

PROPERTIES: calming, purifying

GREAT FOR: massage, bath, cleaning

WHY I LOVE IT: it reminds me of a Thai spa

BLENDS WELL WITH: rosemary, eucalyptus, geranium

Peppermint

PROPERTIES: stimulating, cooling

GREAT FOR: haircare, massage, travel, focus

WHY I LOVE IT: it instantly wakes me up

BLENDS WELL WITH: lemon, grapefruit, sweet orange

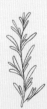

Rosemary

PROPERTIES: stimulating, refreshing

GREAT FOR: haircare, travel, focus

WHY I LOVE IT: it gives me full, healthy brows

BLENDS WELL WITH: lemon, spruce, lavender

Tea tree

PROPERTIES: antibacterial, astringent

GREAT FOR: skincare, cleaning

WHY I LOVE IT: it's earthy and makes cleaning a breeze

BLENDS WELL WITH: sweet orange, lavender, lemon

WOODSY

Cedarwood

PROPERTIES: astringent, warming

GREAT FOR: haircare, shower, cleaning

WHY I LOVE IT: it's incredibly cozy and warm

BLENDS WELL WITH: lavender, bergamot, spruce

Frankincense

PROPERTIES: toning, grounding

GREAT FOR: skincare, meditation, yoga

WHY I LOVE IT: it's a staple in my skincare routine

BLENDS WELL WITH: lavender, bergamot, cedarwood

Spruce

PROPERTIES: purifying, cleansing

GREAT FOR: cleaning, massage, clarity

WHY I LOVE IT: it brings the outdoors inside

BLENDS WELL WITH: eucalyptus, grapefruit, frankincense

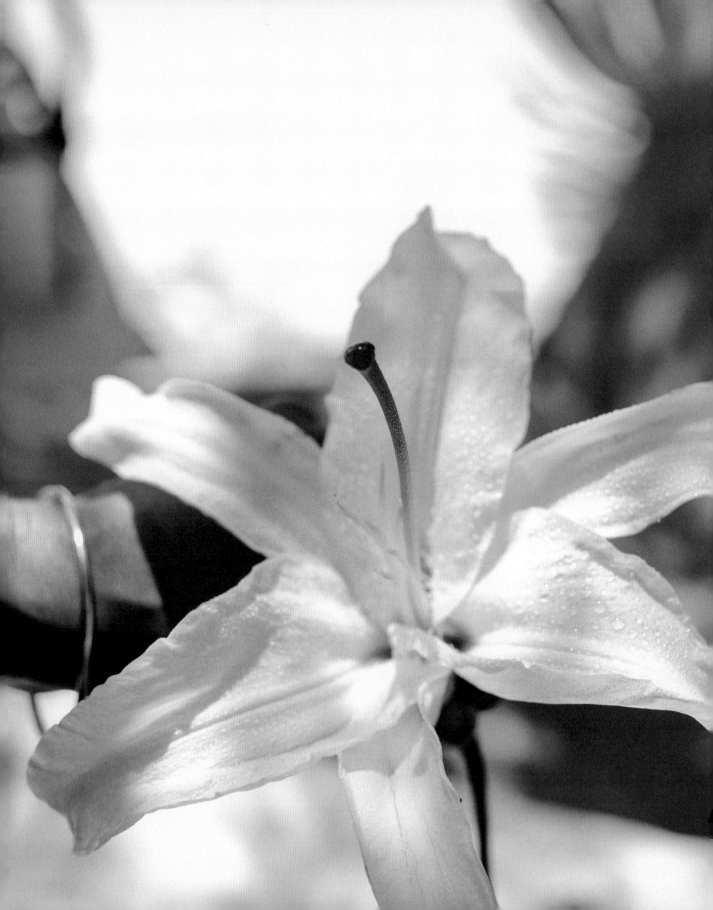

BEAUTY

At first glance, you may think that essential oils are newcomers to the mainstream beauty industry. Perhaps you've noticed that more and more retailers are starting to introduce them to their beauty and wellness departments. Although this development may seem novel to us, the use of essential oils in beauty routines is nothing new at all. Thousands of years ago, in ancient civilizations like those in Egypt, Greece, Rome and India, essential oils were a staple in beauty and hygiene routines. Essential oils like frankincense, myrrh and geranium were incredibly popular and even considered sacred by some. Women like Cleopatra would use essential oils for face oils, steams and body scrubs and as a natural perfume. Luckily for us, their benefits are still very much the same today. On top of all their benefits, what I love about essential oils is thinking about all the women before me who've used them, and how these simple rituals and practices connect us in a small but special way.

The potency and purity of essential oils allow for endless possibilities when it comes to customizing and personalizing your beauty routine. Your skin, hair and nails are always changing and evolving, and I truly believe that your skincare and beauty products should be as dynamic as you are. This chapter will help you navigate the essential oils that are best for your skin—whatever stage it is at. It will also help you create a small bathroom apothecary that will give you the ingredients, recipes and tips to make your own beauty products quickly, easily and cost effectively.

My bathroom apothecary is made up of a few select essential oil bottles and jars that allow me to customize the products I put on my face. These simple practices not only offer great results for my skin, but the act of combining, mixing and customizing a few simple ingredients is also grounding and nourishing for both my skin and my soul. While most of these recipes take only a few short minutes, these practices of self-care act as a reminder for me to slow down and to nurture myself and my well-being, even if it's just for a moment.

DETERMINING YOUR SKIN TYPE "IN THE MOMENT"

I truly believe that your skin is as dynamic as you are—your needs, qualities, moods and priorities change throughout a year, a month, even a day, and shouldn't be pigeon-holed or labelled as a specific personality. It's easy to label your skin as "oily," "dry" or "sensitive," but with so many ongoing changes in your life, it's worth exploring products and recipes for more than one skin type. Long gone are the days when you unconsciously went to the "dry skin" section of the drugstore and picked up a greasy moisturizer. Making your own beauty and skin-care products means that you can meet your skin where it is in that moment, and while it may take a little more time and effort to tune into your needs, the process can start to inspire a lot more than just checking in with your skin. I find that the exercise of thinking of my skin helps prompt me to also think of my own needs as a person and woman. Here are a few ways to guide and help you deter-mine what the needs of your skin are in this moment. Feel free to use them as tools and a reference as you experiment with making new products.

SENSITIVE SKIN

Let's start with a few questions to ask yourself:

- Does my skin get red, itchy or irritated easily?
- Do I get red blotches on my cheeks after exercise or after trying new makeup and skincare products?
- Have I broken out in hives before?

If you answered yes to any of these questions, you may have sensitive skin. Sometimes, during high-stress times in life, our skin can become more reac-tive and sensitive. I find this happens with my own skin, almost as if it's reacting to the business and hustle of life at that time.

Despite popular belief, sensitive skin doesn't have to be high maintenance. If you find that your skin is easily irritated, I recommend sticking to very mild daily cleansing in both the morning and the evening. Other simple rituals, such as aromatic face steaming and masks that are moisturizing and cooling, can be helpful when your skin is feeling super sensitive or inflamed. I also suggest sleeping on soft silk, organic cotton or bamboo sheets and pillowcases—your skin and your overall well-being will thank you. Lastly, it doesn't hurt to use

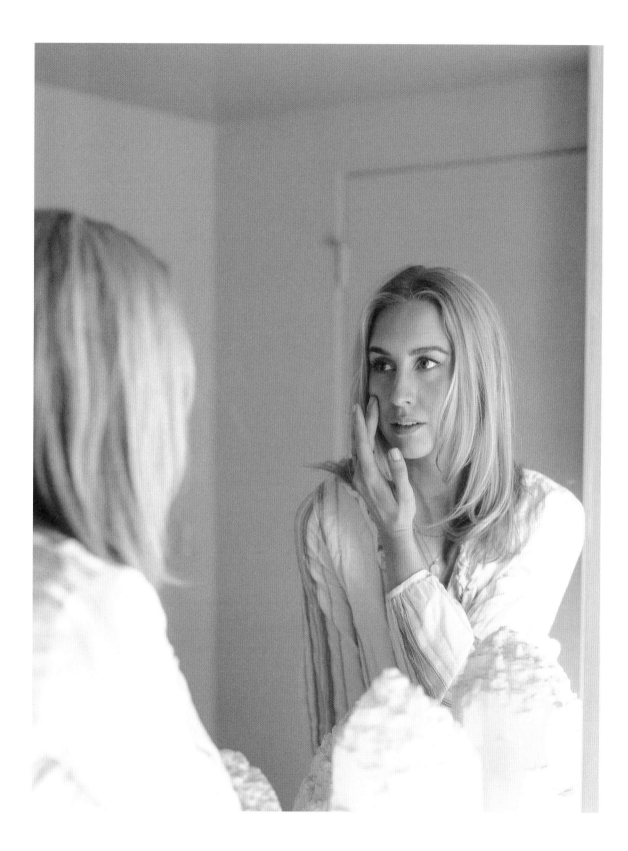

mild natural detergents in your laundry, just to make sure your skin isn't rubbing against unnecessary chemicals.

If you find that your skin is sensitive right now, keep the products you use simple and use the recipes in this book to create your own simple custom home and beauty products. The good news is that they'll be free of any chemicals or synthetics that could contribute to inflammation and irritation.

DRY SKIN

Let's start with a few questions to ask yourself:

- Does my face sting when I apply moisturizer?
- Do I need a cream cleanser instead of gel or soap?
- Does my skin flake if I use face powder?
- Do my lips get chapped easily?

If you answered yes to any of these questions, your skin might be dry. This could be due to diet, genetics or even the weather. Caring for dry skin can be very similar to how you care for sensitive skin. If you have dry skin, avoid skincare products with too many active ingredients, as they can sting the small cuts and irritations that can occur in those with severely dry skin.

Dry skin can be tough, especially in the winter, but achieving that dewy glow can actually be quite simple. I find that most dry skin can benefit from daily cleansing in the morning and evening. A soft and gentle exfoliation twice a week is a nice added touch, especially when paired with aromatic face steaming and moisturizing masks. I'd also recommend gently massaging your face with a jade roller or your fingers while applying cleanser, serum or moisturizer to encourage your skin to create its own natural oils (plus, it feels amazing).

Oil-based skincare products (like the ones found in this book) are especially beneficial for those with dry skin because they help sink right into the dermis of the skin—moisturizing at a deeper level than a greasy topical cream.

OILY SKIN

Let's start with a few questions to ask yourself:

- Do I have oily patches on my skin?
- If I press a tissue on my face, does oil mark the tissue?
- Does my makeup cake easily?
- Do I feel the need to reapply powder or wipe my face throughout the day?

If you answered yes to any of these questions, your skin may be oily. While it may seem counterintuitive to add oils to oily skin, doing so actually has a positive effect. If you're worried about shine and tend to shy away from oil products, your skin is forced to produce more of its own oil. It's a bit of a catch-22.

For oily skin, I suggest a regular skincare regimen that involves clay masks, gentle daily cleansing and a simple daily exfoliation practice that helps unclog pores (without overly drying the skin). Just be cautious not to exfoliate too often, as doing so can dry out the skin and increase oil production further.

Although all the products in this book are made with oil bases, some oils have gentle astringent properties that can help control oil production while keeping the skin moisturized and nourished.

COMBINATION SKIN

Let's start with a few questions to ask yourself:

- Do I have oil around my nose and forehead?
- Does the skin on my cheek feel drier than the skin around my nose?
- Do I find it hard to find a moisturizer that fits my needs?

If you answered yes to any of these questions, you may have combination skin. Being aware of the changing needs of your combination skin is important because it can easily switch from oily to dry—or hey, maybe you even experience both at the same time. If you find that your skin flip-flops frequently, creating custom essential oil skincare products can be a great solution.

For combination skin, I recommend simple daily facial massages while you cleanse and moisturize. Simple toning masks are also great for combination skin, as is finding a simple skincare system that doesn't leave your skin overly hydrated, too dry or irritated.

Most of the recipes in this book will work great for combination skin because all the products come from a place of wanting to create harmony in the skin. The ultimate goal with customized skincare is to achieve balance and deep nourishment, which is a great strategy for combination skin.

MATURE SKIN

Let's start with a few questions to ask yourself:

- Do I have a few decades' worth of stories to tell?
- Does my skin drink up hydration and enjoy being nourished?
- Do I have lines and sunspots from adventures and time spent outside?

If you answered yes to any of these questions, you may have mature skin. While some people start to add products like eye creams, toners, deep evening moisturizers and brightening creams as their skin matures, I believe you can start to simplify your routine. Whatever your age, I recommend a low-maintenance and hydrating skincare routine for mature skin—one that includes oils that are rich in essential fatty acids and nourishing and calming to the skin. Hydrating masks made with natural products, as well as moisturizing serums applied with a facial massage or rollers, can be a nice addition to your routine as well. As far as cleansing goes, I suggest cleansing only in the evening, as the priority is maintaining moisture and avoiding making your skin overly dry.

Your face should have stories to tell—it's seen places, heard stories and faced the world for decades more than most. That's something to celebrate, and creating luxurious and hydrating products is a beautiful reward for that journey. I hope you experiment with the different recipes in this book and put your own spin on them.

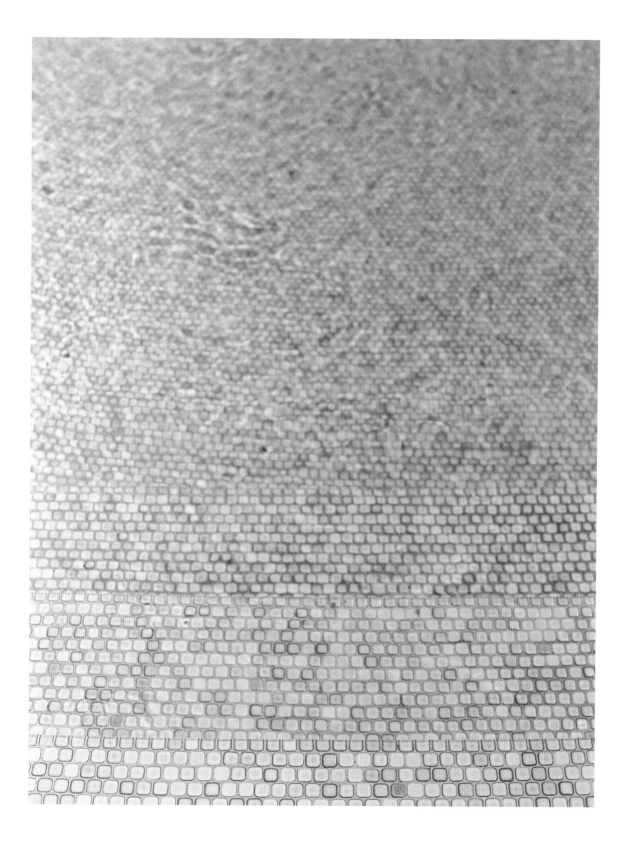

FACE OIL BLENDING GUIDE

What makes oils so exciting is also the same thing that can make them over-whelming. There are so many different essential oils that trying to navigate all their properties and figuring out which ones are best for your skin can make the whole process daunting. Before diving in and creating your own beauty products, take a few short minutes to think intentionally about your skin and what it needs based on its hydration, elasticity, oil levels and moisture levels. This section helps explain which oils and combinations of oils will be best for your skin and beauty routine. Keep in mind that our skin changes, so your use of this section will likely change and evolve with time.

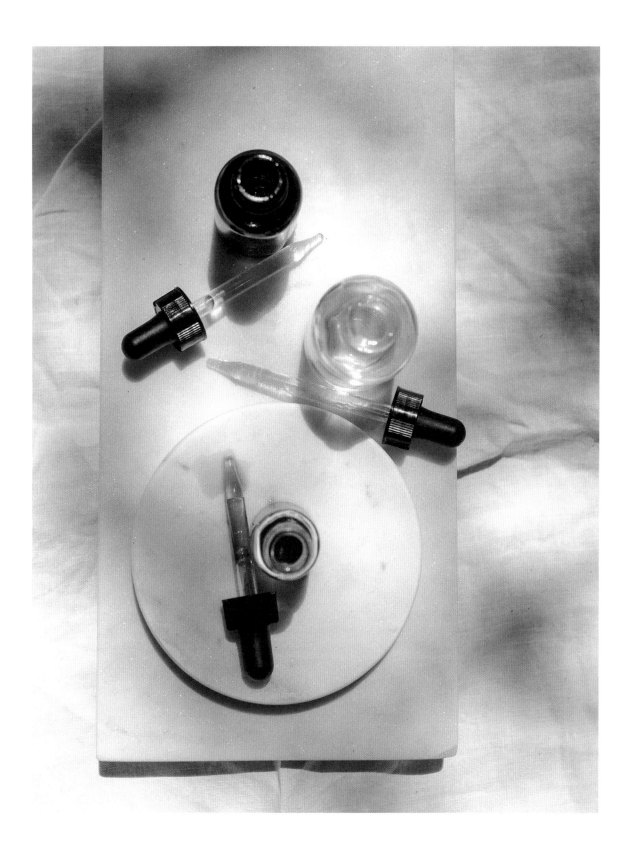

THE THREE COMPONENTS OF A FACE OIL

To create a customized face oil, you need three key components: base oils, complex oils and essential oils. Each provides different benefits, and by combining all three, you're creating a product that's personalized to the needs of your skin.

The first step is choosing your base oil, which will provide the moisturizing level necessary for your skin. Next, you'll decide which combination of complex oils you'd like to add—these will add more specific benefits to the skin based on your needs, such as toning or adding antioxidants. The final step is choosing the essential oils. The essential oils give the face oil an aroma, and they function as the last step in customizing your product by including oils with astringent, balancing or even brightening qualities. I've outlined the three-step process in a little more detail below.

1. CHOOSE YOUR BASE OIL
Your base oil will help address the moisture level you're looking for based on your skin type. It also makes up the largest portion of the face oil mixture. You can think of it as the "vessel" that carries your complex oils and essential oils into the skin while giving you the hydration and moisturizing level you need. To start formulating your face oil, consider whether you need an oil that's a little richer and stays hydrating for longer or something lighter that sinks into the skin quickly without lingering or leaving residue.

2. CHOOSE YOUR COMPLEX OILS
Complex oils have more nutrients and do more "work" for the skin than a base oil. I choose complex oils that are specific to the needs of my skin on any given day—whether that be dullness, severe dryness or fine lines due to fatigue and not drinking enough water.

3. CHOOSE YOUR ESSENTIAL OILS
The last step in creating your own custom face oil is adding your essential oils. These oils make up the smallest quantity of the mixture, but they have strong benefits and also add scent to your creation. If you're extremely sensitive to fragrance, you can opt out of this part, but most of these oils are gentle enough that they shouldn't cause irritation. Again, remember to choose oils that address the needs of your skin type and have the properties you're looking for.

CHOOSING YOUR OILS BY SKIN TYPE

Think of this section as a cheat sheet that can help you determine which specific base, complex, and essential oils you'll want to use based on the needs of your skin. Remember that you can absolutely experiment within the different skin types, as these notes are just suggestions. Who knows, you may find something that works brilliantly for your skin, even if it doesn't fall under your "skin type."

SENSITIVE SKIN

BASE OILS FOR SENSITIVE SKIN

Apricot kernel oil
A moisturizing yet gentle oil for the skin that's particularly nice to use in the evening.

Grapeseed oil
An ultra-light oil that sinks into the skin quickly and won't appear greasy. It's great for those who have nut allergies, too.

Jojoba oil
A very nourishing oil that sinks into the skin quickly because it mimics the oils naturally found in the skin.

COMPLEX OILS FOR SENSITIVE SKIN

Blueberry seed oil
A powerful antioxidant, this oil can be used in small quantities for sensitive skin to help build strength and help repair stressed skin.

Rosehip oil
Rosehip oil is a great choice for sensitive skin because it has super gentle reparative qualities and can help calm redness.

ESSENTIAL OILS FOR SENSITIVE SKIN

Chamomile essential oil
The most gentle essential oil, it's especially great for creating evening beauty products thanks to its natural sedative qualities.

Geranium essential oil
Geranium oil can help balance the skin's pH while also helping to decrease redness and inflammation.

Lavender essential oil
With soothing properties, lavender can help calm down inflammatory skin.

DRY SKIN

BASE OILS FOR DRY SKIN

Avocado oil
Avocado oil is an excellent source of antioxidants and essential fatty acids. It's very nourishing and also soothing for the skin, which makes it helpful for those with flaky or severely dry skin.

Hemp seed oil
With a high percentage of omega-3 and omega-6 fatty acids, hemp oil has a composition similar to skin's natural lipids, which means it sinks into the skin as a very effective moisturizer for those with dry skin.

Plum Oil
Plum is a super luxurious, rich oil that's great for dry skin because it's packed with omegas. It also smells heavenly.

COMPLEX OILS FOR DRY SKIN

Meadowfoam seed oil
A hydrating oil that helps lock moisture into the skin. It's great to combine with other oils to trap the benefits of essential oils.

Pomegranate seed oil
A thick, replenishing oil that's very gentle on the skin. It creates a moisturizing, protective shield, which makes it great for overnight facial treatments.

Rosehip oil
An oil that's packed with vitamins, antioxidants and essential fatty acids that are known to help improve the hydration of dry or itchy skin. It's also helpful for preventing fine lines, which can be more common with dry skin.

ESSENTIAL OILS FOR DRY SKIN

Cedarwood essential oil
A woodsy essential oil that can help decrease signs of irritation caused by dryness.

Frankincense essential oil
Harvested as a resin from a tree, this essential oil is very nourishing and hydrating for the skin, which can decrease flaking and extreme dryness.

Ylang ylang essential oil

Nourishing and gentle, ylang ylang is great for both aging and dry skin. It's especially helpful around the eye area and anywhere where lines and dryness are showing up.

OILY SKIN

BASE OILS FOR OILY SKIN

Apricot kernel oil

A moisturizing yet gentle oil for the skin that's particularly nice to use in the evening.

Grapeseed oil

An ultra-light oil that sinks into the skin quickly and will not appear greasy. It's great for morning face oil blends because you can apply your makeup over it if needed.

COMPLEX OILS FOR OILY SKIN

Raspberry seed oil

An oil that's rich in essential fatty acids and has very high levels of vitamin E, which act as antioxidants, and vitamin A. It's light and pairs well with citrus essential oils, which can be nice to use with oil-prone skin.

Rosehip oil

Very light and delicate, this oil sinks quickly into the skin yet provides essential fatty acids needed to nourish the skin.

Sea buckthorn oil

A slightly astringent oil known for its bright red and orange hue, sea buckthorn oil also provides nourishing properties that help rejuvenate the skin.

ESSENTIAL OILS FOR OILY SKIN

Grapefruit essential oil

A fresh and slightly astringent essential oil that helps freshen and uplift oily skin. It's best used in the evening because it's photosensitive and should not be applied to the skin during prolonged direct sun exposure.

Lavender essential oil

Lavender has gentle antimicrobial and antibacterial properties and is slightly astringent, which makes it a nice choice for people with oily skin or sensitive skin that's prone to being more oily.

Tea tree essential oil

A strong astringent essential oil, tea tree is best known for helping with controlling bacteria in the pores, which can help those who are prone to blemishes or clogged pores.

COMBINATION SKIN

BASE OILS FOR COMBINATION SKIN

Apricot kernel oil

A good "happy medium" oil that's moisturizing and gentle for the skin. It's particularly nice to use in the evening.

Sweet almond oil

A nice, mild all-seasons oil that helps balance dry patches in combination skin, while not overly moisturizing the more oily areas.

COMPLEX OILS FOR COMBINATION SKIN

Evening primrose oil

Evening primrose is a gentle oil with balancing qualities that can help address hormone and stress-related skin changes.

Sea buckthorn oil

Sea buckthorn oil is great for combination skin because it's nourishing and slightly astringent at the same time.

ESSENTIAL OILS FOR COMBINATION SKIN

Grapefruit essential oil

The incredibly fresh and uplifting aroma of grapefruit essential oil is a nice balance between acting as hydration and an astringent for combination skin.

Lavender essential oil

Calming yet effective, lavender oil can help soothe inflammation and redness while also offering gentle antimicrobial and antibacterial properties, which makes it helpful for oil-prone areas of the face.

MATURE SKIN

BASE OILS FOR MATURE SKIN

Hemp seed oil
Hemp seed oil is great for mature skin because it has natural healing properties that deeply hydrate skin that's seen a lot of sun or been exposed to the elements. It's also non-comedogenic, so it won't clog any pores.

Plum oil
Ultra-hydrating, plum oil is great for mature skin because of its plumping qualities. It's great for evening face oils when you want to wake up feeling nourished with a natural glow.

COMPLEX OILS FOR MATURE SKIN

Blueberry seed oil
Blueberry seed oil is wonderful for mature skin because it has antioxidant and repairing qualities that make it beneficial for skin that has been exposed to more sun and adventures.

Evening primrose oil
A standard great choice for mature skin, evening primrose oil helps support skin that's experiencing changes due to hormones and provides a high level of antioxidants.

Meadowfoam seed oil
A favourite oil for mature skin because it provides intense moisture and helps replenish the skin to feel pillowy soft.

ESSENTIAL OILS FOR MATURE SKIN

Frankincense essential oil
A resinous oil that's deeply hydrating and has been used for centuries to promote youthful, healthy-looking skin.

Ylang ylang essential oil
A favourite oil for mature skin, ylang ylang oil has a thick, sap-like consistency and extremely strong floral aroma. It's great for use around the eye and in areas where lines form.

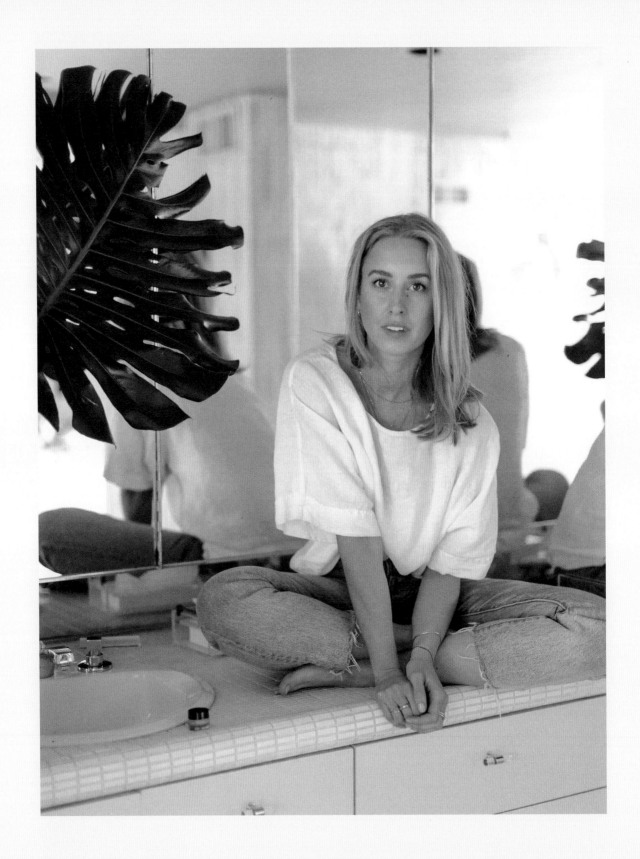

MORNING BEAUTY RITUALS

Although mornings can be hectic, they can also be one of the best times to experiment with new routines and rituals. Often when we think of morning rituals, we think of squeezing in a quick workout or a few moments of meditation or trying a new smoothie recipe. But for me, some of my favourite ways to start my mornings involve incredibly simple and easy wellness-centric beauty rituals. Most of these practices take less than 3 minutes and leave me feeling a little more centred and goddess-like after looking at my inbox and schedule for the day. By carving out a few minutes in your morning to try one of these nourishing recipes, you can start the day knowing you've taken a bit of time for your own wellness before you take on the day and whatever life may bring you.

My suggestion is to try one or two of the following morning rituals each week and then see which ones fit best into your lifestyle at that particular time. It's important to remember that the needs of your skin are dynamic and changing. They change seasonally as well as with fluctuating stress levels, hormones, travel or general life changes. Seeing these rituals as touchpoints and resources for your own wellness make them a great exercise in listening to your skin, hair and nails and determining how you can best nourish yourself.

QUICK FACE STEAMS

You don't need to book a spa appointment or professional facial to enjoy the benefits of a face steam. This easy 10-second, at-home treatment opens the pores and cleanses the skin deeper than an average cleansing would. It's one of my favourite ways to create a spa experience to start off my day—any day of the week.

For me, beginning my day with one of these simple 10-second face steams is an easy luxury that elevates the usual routine of splashing water on my face. I cleanse my face gently and then layer a warm face cloth on it and allow the steam to remove any dirt and residue from the evening prior. By removing all the residue, this technique primes the skin, leaving you with a clean slate and open pores, so that your toners, serums and moisturizers can work more effectively. These quick face steams are a great way to stimulate the senses using essential oils and aromas, while also creating a sense of ritual at the beginning of each day.

Each quick face steam incorporates a breathing meditation, which allows you to experience two rituals at once. The intention is that it will leave both your face and your heart glowing. This breathing exercise is something I do every morning, regardless of where I am in the world or how long the to-do list that awaits me.

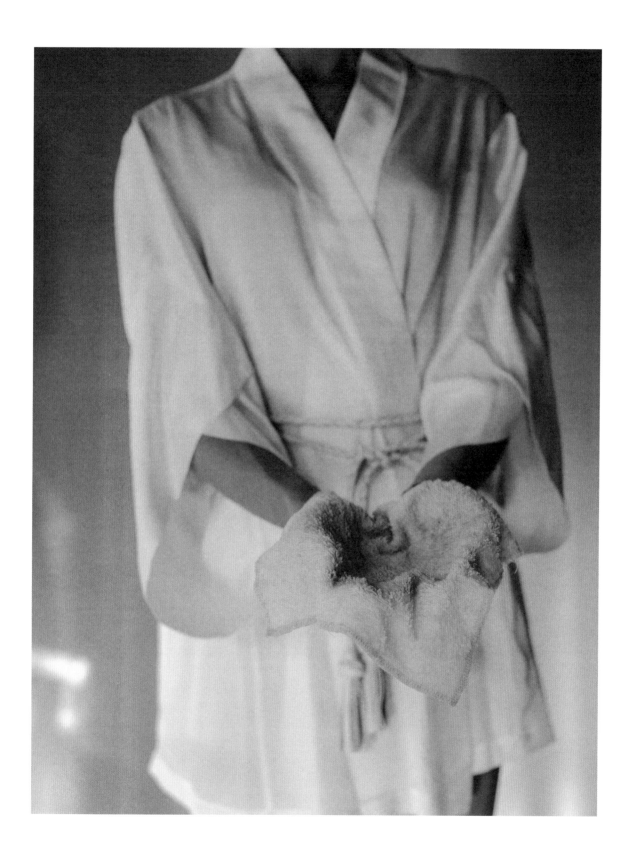

Brightening Face Steam

Not a morning person? Cue this uplifting, citrusy face steam.

TIME: 5 minutes

MAKES: 1 face steam

YOU'LL NEED: a face cloth

COMPONENTS

2 drops grapefruit essential oil

2 drops sweet orange essential oil

1 drop lemon essential oil

If you're looking for something to naturally wake up your skin, citrus aromas are always a safe bet—they have a natural morning vibe. This blend, in particular, gives off the aroma of freshly squeezed orange juice, which is really the best way to start your day. As for the skin benefits, grapefruit and lemon essential oils have slightly astringent properties, which are nice for toning and tightening the pores before you apply makeup in the morning. Sweet orange essential oil is hydrating, contains the benefits of vitamin C associated with oranges and also breaks down excess oil on the skin. I find this brightening face steam especially beneficial when I'm having trouble adjusting to a new time zone while travelling. The fresh aroma helps me perk up and citrus can help aid nausea experienced after early alarm clocks, wake-up calls from the kids or flights you need to be on before sunrise.

METHOD

1. Run a face cloth under hot water. Wring it out and open it across one hand. With the other hand, apply the essential oils to the face cloth by dotting them randomly on its surface. Then, close the two sides of the face cloth together. The warmth from the hot water will heat the essential oils, which helps disperse the aroma and properties throughout the cloth.

APPLICATION

1. Place the warm cloth over your face while leaving space for your nose to breathe.
2. Close your eyes, take a big inhale through the nose, pause, then exhale. Repeat this breathing sequence 3 times. This may seem like a long time, but if you are like most of us, these will likely be the most present and deepest breaths you take all day—so enjoy. Take this time in the morning to ground your feet on the floor, lengthen your spine and fill yourself up with positivity and motivation for the day. With each exhale, let go of whatever negative thoughts, energy or worries you have about what the day will bring.
3. After your face steam, use the same face cloth to wipe away any excess dirt. If you are applying makeup after, rinse your face with cooler water to ensure the pores are closed. If not, continue with your regular facial routine.

Balancing Face Steam

A face steam for when your skin (or life) feels all over the place.

TIME: 5 minutes

MAKES: 1 face steam

YOU'LL NEED: a face cloth

COMPONENTS

2 drops ylang ylang essential oil

2 drops geranium essential oil

1 drop frankincense essential oil

Some days feel more in the flow than others. There are days when I wake up and it energizes me knowing the schedule, appointments, to-do lists and meetings I have ahead. On the other hand, there are days when the stress of living a full, dynamic life weighs on me a bit. That's when I need tools to help me stay on course, to think clearly and feel grounded and to take time to recharge. When I'm not recharged, this feeling of depletion shows up on my face, whether in dry patches, oils spots, or a feeling of congestion. I turn to this balancing face steam on the mornings when I know there is a lot coming at me and my skin. I hope this recipe provides a reminder at the start of your day to breathe and find small, 10-second moments in your day to come back to the centre.

Ylang ylang is a beautiful feminine flower that makes a thick, almost sap-like essential oil. Given its potent floral aroma, only a small amount is needed to enjoy its benefits. Geranium essential oil is one of my personal favourites because it has the balancing benefits of a floral essential oil but also a slightly herbal, minty undertone that refreshes and tones the skin. I also add a small drop of frankincense essential oil to this morning face steam because it has restorative qualities, which is a nice way to start the day.

METHOD

1. Run a face cloth under hot water. Wring it out and open it across one hand. With the other hand, apply the essential oils to the face cloth by dotting them randomly on its surface. Then, close the two sides of the face cloth together. The warmth from the hot water will heat the essential oils, which helps disperse the aroma and properties throughout the cloth.

APPLICATION

1. Place the warm cloth over your face while leaving space for your nose to breathe.
2. Close your eyes, take a big inhale through the nose, pause, then exhale. Repeat this breathing sequence 3 times. This may seem like a long time, but if you are like most of us, these will likely be the most present and deepest breaths you take all day—so enjoy. Take this time in the morning to ground your feet on the floor, lengthen your spine and fill yourself up with positivity and motivation for the day. With each exhale, let go of whatever negative thoughts, energy or worries you have about what the day will bring.
3. After your face steam, use the same face cloth to wipe away any excess dirt. If you are applying makeup after, rinse your face with cooler water to ensure the pores are closed. If not, continue with your regular facial routine.

Clarifying Face Steam

A face steam for when that blemish pops up out of literally nowhere.

TIME: 5 minutes

MAKES: 1 face steam

YOU'LL NEED: a face cloth

COMPONENTS

3 drops lavender essential oil

2 drops tea tree essential oil

Some days I wake up with the feeling that a blemish is about to appear, or worse . . . it already has. To nip this in the bud, I usually turn to a deep cleanse of the pores. I find that a clarifying face steam is more effective than just cleansing and applying a blemish spot treatment. I tend to do this treatment if I'm travelling and there's more pollution in the air (hello, NYC in the summer) or if I'm feeling congestion on my face from not eating enough greens or not drinking enough water.

This clarifying face steam should be used when your skin needs a really deep clean. Take note that it's especially important to keep your eyes closed while applying the cloth over your face because the volatile oils from tea tree essential oil can be intense and sting the eyes. Lavender essential oil has similar properties to tea tree essential oil in that it really gets into the pores and has natural antibacterial properties. Both of these oils can help with decreasing the tendency to get blemishes caused by bacteria or clogged pores. The aroma of this face steam reminds me of an intensive spa treatment; the lavender essential oil is calming, while the tea tree essential oil is fresh and clean. It's the perfect reset to start the day.

METHOD
1. Run a face cloth under hot water. Wring it out and open it across one hand. With the other hand, apply the essential oils to the face cloth by dotting them randomly on its surface. Then, close the two sides of the face cloth together. The warmth from the hot water will heat the essential oils, which helps disperse the aroma and properties throughout the cloth.

APPLICATION
1. Place the warm cloth over your face while leaving space to breathe through your nose.
2. Close your eyes, take a big inhale through the nose, pause, and exhale. Repeat this breathing sequence 3 times. This may seem like a long time, but if you are like most of us, these will likely be the most present and deepest breaths you take all day—so enjoy. Take this time in the morning to ground your feet on the floor, lengthen your spine and fill yourself up with positivity and motivation for the day. With each exhale, let go of whatever negative thoughts, energy or worries you have about what the day will bring.
3. After your face steam, use the same face cloth to wipe away any excess dirt. If you are applying makeup after, rinse your face with cooler water to ensure the pores are closed. If not, continue with your regular facial routine.

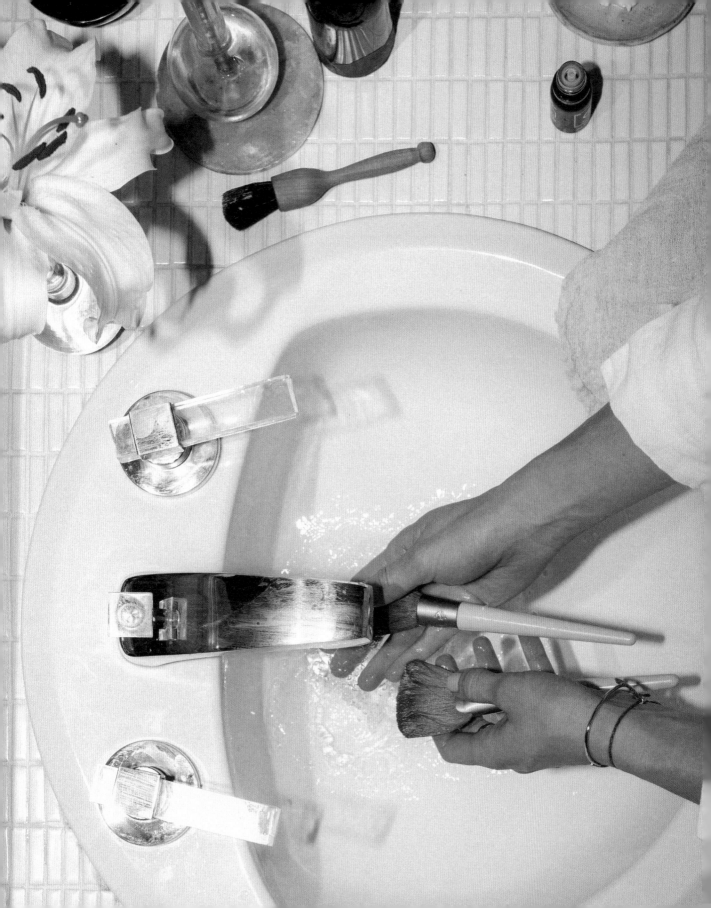

MORNING FACE OIL CLEANSERS

Using a gentle oil cleanser is my favourite way to wash my face. Cleansing with oil might sound counterintuitive at first, but oil cleansers actually can be more effective and are more nourishing to the skin than a soap-based, astringent cleanser. Even for those with oily skin, oil cleansers are a great treatment. When paired with the correct essential oils, they provide properties that help your brain and skin wake up naturally.

Each of these morning face oil cleansers is designed for the dynamic needs of your skin. When we have jam-packed schedules or are overwhelmed by the modern hustle, it's easy to forget to check in with ourselves each morning. Using customized facial products can act as a great reminder to do just that. I find this cleansing ritual a simple way to carve out time for myself to take a deep breath and check in with myself. Who would have thought a face cleansing oil could mean so much?

These cleansers can be made ahead of time (I like making mine on a Sunday afternoon), and the quantity should last you a week or two. You can also halve the recipes or make them in much smaller amounts daily if you want to customize the cleanser each morning. It really depends on the time you have and the systems and recipes you find work best for your skin. I suggest making a few smaller batches of these different combinations and then finding the one that's best for your skin at this phase in your life. I usually make enough to last me 2 weeks at a time because . . . life.

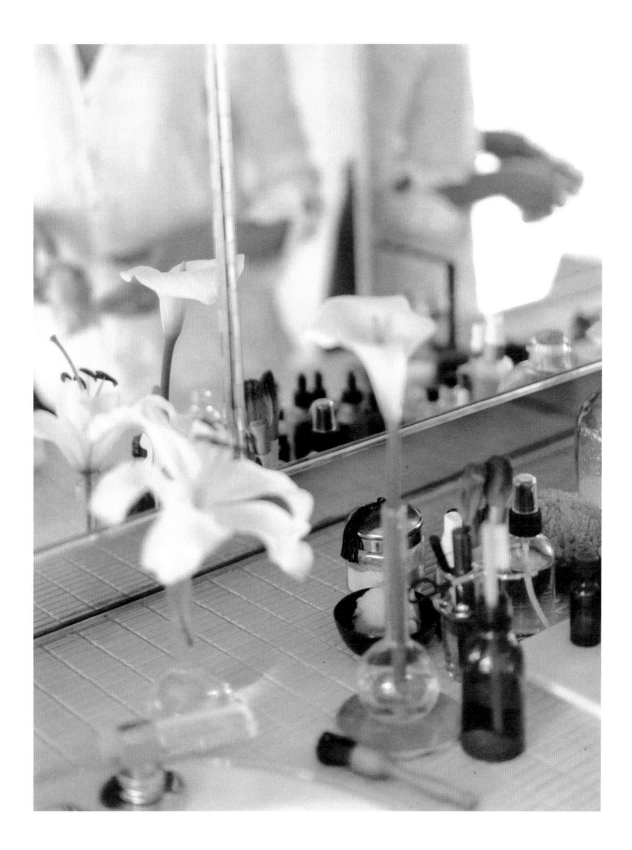

Energizing Face Oil Cleanser

An oil cleanser for when your face needs a pick-me-up.

TIME: 10 minutes

MAKES: 1 ounce (30 mL) face cleanser

YOU'LL NEED: a small bowl and a face cloth

COMPONENTS

1 tablespoon organic solid virgin coconut oil

1 tablespoon grapeseed oil

2 drops geranium essential oil

1 drop sweet orange essential oil

1 drop grapefruit essential oil

I use this energizing face cleansing oil when my skin looks as tired as I feel (which is most mornings before drinking an espresso). I enjoy using this as an everyday cleanser because the properties of coconut oil are naturally anti-bacterial, which helps prevent blemishes. Sweet orange and grapefruit essential oils are perfect for morning cleansers because of their tendency to be uplifting and refreshing. Plus, their strong citrus aromas give off energized morning vibes. Geranium essential oil is a nice addition to this blend because of its balancing effects on the skin, and it has a slightly minty floral aroma, which adds a feminine freshness.

METHOD

1. In a small bowl, mix together all components until smooth with a paste-like consistency. If the coconut oil is in a fully solid state, you may need to warm the bowl with your hands or heat the coconut oil slightly by running the coconut oil jar under hot water.

APPLICATION

1. Using your fingers, massage 1 to 2 teaspoons of the face oil cleanser into your face in small upward circles while avoiding the eyes.
2. While massaging your face, take 3 deep breaths in through your nose and out through your mouth, pausing in between each breath for the count of 2. During this time, you can also experiment with massaging areas of tension displayed on the facial pressure point illustration (page 47).
3. When done, use a warm, damp face cloth to wipe away any excess oil cleanser. Then place the face cloth over your face (leaving space for your nose) and take 3 more deep breaths while pressing the face cloth gently into your face.
4. Wipe away any remaining face oil cleanser and then follow with the toner and/or moisturizer of your choice.

STORAGE

Keep in a cool, dry place away from direct sunlight for up to 1 week.

Restorative Face Oil Cleanser

An oil cleanser for when your skin needs a little extra TLC.

TIME: 10 minutes

MAKES: 1 ounce (30 mL) face cleanser

YOU'LL NEED: a small bowl and a face cloth

COMPONENTS

1 tablespoon organic solid virgin coconut oil

1 tablespoon jojoba oil

1 drop ylang ylang essential oil

1 drop lemongrass essential oil

1 drop frankincense essential oil

This restorative morning face cleansing oil is my favourite cleanser to use on the weekend or while travelling—basically, any time my skin needs to recharge and experience some extra attention and hydration. The essential oils used in this cleansing blend are balancing and nourishing, and the base oils are some of the most moisturizing ones you can find. Jojoba oil is used for this cleansing oil because it closely mimics the oil naturally found in our skin, which means it sinks into the skin while cleansing and leaves the skin feeling nourished and not depleted or dry like a soap-based cleanser would. Adding hydration while cleansing helps restore moisture and fullness to the skin, which is especially important for tired or dehydrated skin.

This cleansing oil is a lifesaver for dry skin in the winter months (it holds up against cold Canadian winters) as well as when travelling—especially by plane, which can easily dehydrate the skin.

METHOD

1. In a small bowl, mix together all components until smooth with a paste-like consistency. If the coconut oil is in a fully solid state, you may need to warm the bowl with your hands or heat the coconut oil slightly by running the coconut oil jar under hot water.

APPLICATION

1. Using your fingers, massage 1 to 2 teaspoons of the face oil cleanser into your face in small upward circles while avoiding the eyes.
2. While massaging your face, take 3 deep breaths in through your nose and out through your mouth, pausing in between each breath for the count of 2. During this time, you can also experiment with massaging areas of tension displayed on the facial pressure point illustration (page 47).
3. When done, use a warm, damp face cloth to wipe away any excess oil cleanser. Then place the face cloth over your face (leaving space for your nose) and take 3 more deep breaths while pressing the face cloth gently into your face.
4. Wipe away any remaining face oil cleanser and then follow with the toner and/or moisturizer of your choice.

STORAGE

Keep in a cool, dry place away from direct sunlight for up to 1 week.

Calming Face Oil Cleanser

An oil cleanser for when your skin (or mind) needs soothing.

TIME: 10 minutes

MAKES: 1.5 ounces (45 mL) face cleanser

YOU'LL NEED: a small bowl and a face cloth

COMPONENTS

1 tablespoon organic solid virgin coconut oil

1 tablespoon organic full-fat canned coconut milk

1 tablespoon grapeseed oil

1 drop lavender essential oil (optional)

This simple and very pure face oil cleanser can be used daily if you have sensitive skin, or when your skin is feeling irritated. I tend to use this calming face oil cleanser after eating too much sugar or indulging in one too many glasses of wine. I've also used it while travelling after my skin reacted from using hotel face cloths and sheets that were cleaned with a harsh laundry detergent. This calming cleanser is a great tool to have in your bathroom during the summer months, too. If your skin is feeling sensitive from excess heat and sun exposure, this soothing ritual will do just the trick.

METHOD

1. In a small bowl, mix together all components until smooth with a paste-like consistency. If the coconut oil is in a fully solid state, you may need to warm the bowl with your hands or heat the coconut oil slightly by running the coconut oil jar under hot water.

APPLICATION

1. Using your fingers, massage about 1 teaspoon of the face oil cleanser into your face in small upward circles while avoiding the eyes.
2. While massaging your face, take 3 deep breaths in through your nose and out through your mouth, pausing in between each breath for the count of 2. During this time, you can also experiment with massaging areas of tension displayed on the facial pressure point illustration (page 47).
3. When done, use a warm, damp face cloth to wipe away any excess oil cleanser. Then place the face cloth over your face (leaving space for your nose) and take 3 more deep breaths while pressing the face cloth gently into your face.
4. Wipe away any remaining face oil cleanser and then follow with the toner and/or moisturizer of your choice.

STORAGE

Keep in a cool, dry place for up to 1 week. I like to keep mine in the fridge so that it feels extra soothing and calming when applied.

FACIAL PRESSURE POINT MASSAGE

I love creating small moments to recharge and re-centre. One way to do this is by adding a facial pressure point massage into your face oil, serum or cleansing routine. This will help relieve tension that can often be stored around the eyes, jaw and cheeks.

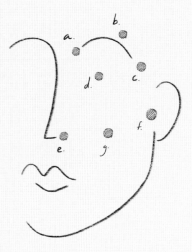

STEPS

1. Make sure your hands are washed and clean. Place a few drops of your desired face oil, serum or cleanser into the palms and gently rub the palms together.
2. Cup the hands over the mouth and nose and gently inhale for the benefits of the aroma before the pressure point massage.

EYE AREA PRESSURE POINTS

Using your ring fingers, press lightly at the inner eyebrows. Then press lightly at the middle of the eyebrow, on each temple, and beneath the middle of the eye area on the top of the cheekbone directly under the pupil. Hold each point for 2 to 3 seconds and breathe deeply.

a. Inner eye socket at the start of the brow: can help decrease tension related to eye strain.
b. Mid eyebrow: can help relieve tension related to the sinuses.
c. Temples: can help decrease tension stored in the head related to stress.
d. Under eyes: can help relieve eye pressure from too many hours at a computer screen.

NOSE PRESSURE POINT

e. Using your ring fingers, press at either side of the nostril. Hold for 2 to 3 seconds and breathe deeply.

CHEEKBONE PRESSURE POINTS

Using your ring fingers, press where the jawline and cheekbone meet (it should line up with the middle of the ear). Hold for 2 to 3 seconds and breathe deeply. Then move to the centre of the cheekbone and hold for 2 to 3 seconds.

f. Jawline at cheekbone: can help relieve tension in the jaw from clenching.
g. Middle cheekbone: can help relieve tension in the cheeks.

BOTANICAL FACE TONERS

Toning is an essential yet often overlooked step in a skincare routine. The purpose of using a toner in the morning is to add a layer of hydration before sealing in that hydration with a moisturizer. In the past, toners have been marketed for oily skin because low-quality, commercial skincare has popularized astringent and alcohol-based toners as ways to control and prevent oil production. This isn't what you want for your skin; a toner shouldn't be drying. It should be used to help refresh, nourish, hydrate and balance the skin's pH after cleansing. It should also remove any leftover dirt and makeup that was not removed during cleansing.

These botanical face toners are super easy to make, and you can switch up which ones you're using depending on your skin type at that moment. These are great for mornings or evenings and should be made in small batches and kept in the fridge or a cool, dark place to enhance their soothing or cooling properties. I prefer to use a filtered or distilled water base for toners.

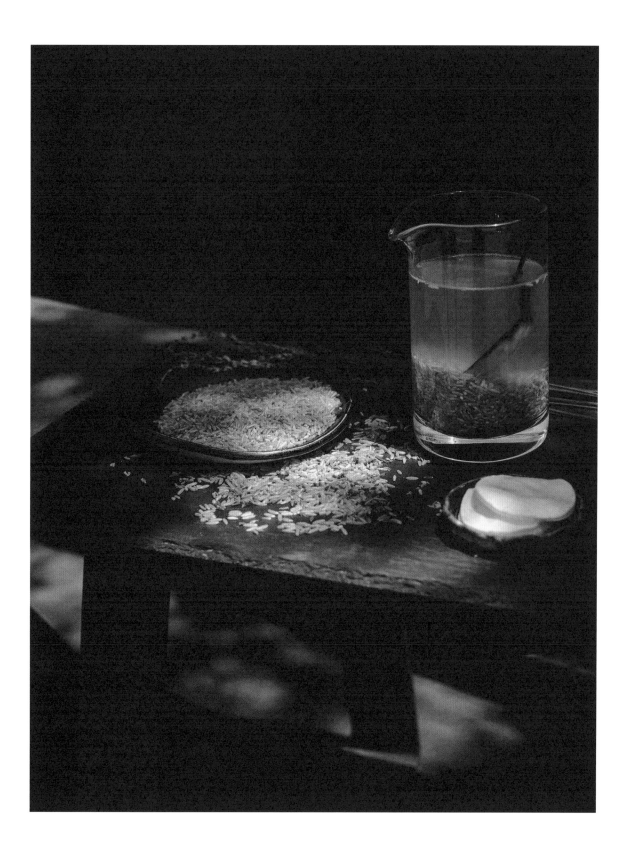

Rice Water Lavender Face Toner (Sensitive Skin)

A delicate, refreshing face toner that uses ingredients from your pantry.

TIME: 30 minutes

MAKES: 8 ounces (240 mL) toner

YOU'LL NEED: a 16-ounce (480 mL) jar or bowl, an 8-ounce (240 mL) mist bottle and 3 organic cotton face pads

COMPONENTS

½ cup organic white or brown rice

1 cup filtered water

5 drops lavender essential oil

Rice water is an incredibly dynamic and easy-to-make skincare asset that, while not commonly used, has become a staple in my beauty routine. Soaking organic white or brown rice (I prefer brown) in room-temperature filtered water for at least 30 minutes (overnight is even better, if you have time) results in a beautifully soothing and slightly mattifying water. Rice water helps calm and smooth the complexion of the face and neck using the natural enzymes found in rice. Since rice is a grain, the rice water should be kept cool and can last for up to 5 days in the fridge before you need to make a new batch.

METHOD

1. In a jar, add the rice and cover with the filtered water until the water level is 1 inch higher than the rice. This will leave room for the rice to expand naturally while covered by the water. As the rice starts to soak up the water, the liquid should turn cloudy and the rice may start rising to the top of the container. Soak the rice for at least 30 minutes.
2. Drain the cloudy rice water into a mist bottle and discard the rice (or store in the fridge to cook for a healthy snack).
3. Add the lavender essential oil to the rice water, then place a lid on the mist bottle and shake well.

APPLICATION

1. Shake the rice water toner vigorously before using to evenly distribute the lavender essential oil throughout the liquid. It's normal for the oil to separate to the top of the mixture because the toner is completely natural and doesn't contain any toxic emulsifiers or additives.
2. After cleansing the face, mist the toner directly onto 2 cotton face pads.
3. With a damp cotton face pad in each hand, start in the middle of your face and make light downward and outward strokes from the middle of the nose out, from the middle of the forehead out and from the middle of the chin out.
4. Mist the toner directly onto a clean cotton face pad. Using the damp cotton face pad, start at the base of your neck and make light upward strokes toward the jawline.
5. Let the face toner sink into the skin for 10 to 15 seconds, then continue your facial routine. Follow with serum, moisturizer and/or eye creams.

STORAGE

Keep in the fridge for up to 5 days.

Chamomile, Honey and Frankincense Face Toner (Dry Skin)

A toner for when your skin is crying for a little moisture.

TIME: 30 minutes

MAKES: 4.9 ounces (145 mL) face toner

YOU'LL NEED: a 6-ounce (180 mL) mist bottle and 3 organic cotton face pads

COMPONENTS

½ cup boiling filtered water

1 organic chamomile tea bag

1 teaspoon organic liquid honey

1 tablespoon organic apple cider vinegar

1 drop frankincense essential oil

STORAGE

Keep in the fridge for up to 2 weeks.

Toners can seem unnecessary during the winter months or for those with dry skin, but unlike astringent, alcohol-based toners, this natural chamomile and honey–infused toner helps lock in moisture and hydration. When paired with the right oil cleanser and moisturizing oil, it can make a big difference in the hydration level of your skin.

The chamomile tea in this toner helps soothe the skin, which can be irritated when dry, and the honey is added to give the toner a moisturizing quality. The small amount of apple cider vinegar helps provide a gentle astringent effect that isn't drying or irritating to the skin. Note: if the skin on your face is very dry or cracked at all, make this recipe without the apple cider vinegar, as applying it to delicate chapped or cracked skin could be irritating.

METHOD

1. Add the boiling water and chamomile tea bag to a ceramic or heatproof container (a glass jar works just fine) and let steep for 10 minutes. Remove the tea bag and let the tea cool. It's important to let the tea cool fully because if you add essential oils to warm water, the volatile oils will evaporate and you won't get their full benefits.
2. Add the honey, apple cider vinegar and frankincense essential oil to the tea, then stir or shake well to dissolve the honey. Pour the mixture into a mist bottle.

APPLICATION

1. Shake the toner vigorously before using to evenly distribute the honey and frankincense essential oil throughout the liquid. It's normal for the components to separate to the top of the mixture because the toner is completely natural and doesn't contain any toxic emulsifiers or additives.
2. After cleansing the face, mist the toner directly onto 2 cotton face pads.
3. With a damp cotton face pad in each hand, start in the middle of your face and make light downward and outward strokes from the middle of the nose out, from the middle of the forehead out and from the middle of the chin out.
4. Mist the toner directly onto a clean cotton face pad. Using the damp cotton face pad, start at the base of your neck and make light upward strokes toward the jawline.
5. Let the face toner sink into the skin for 10 to 15 seconds, then continue your facial routine. Follow with serum, moisturizer and/or eye creams.

Grapefruit and Green Tea Face Toner (Oily Skin)

A cooling toner for when hormones or travel has your skin hot and bothered.

TIME: 15 minutes

MAKES: 9.9 ounces (295 mL) face toner

YOU'LL NEED: a 12-ounce (360 mL) mist bottle or glass jar with a lid

COMPONENTS

1 cup boiling filtered water

2 organic green tea bags

¼ cup non-alcoholic witch hazel

3 drops grapefruit essential oil

STORAGE

Keep in the fridge for up to 2 weeks.

What I love about this green tea and grapefruit toner is how simple it is to make. It really exemplifies how DIY beauty products can be part of your usual morning routine. For this toner, I use two green tea bags, which I am usually steeping in the morning anyway, and add a few drops of grapefruit essential oil. I also like to have grapefruit essential oil diffusing in the background while I tone, just to round out the experience and boost my morning mood.

So, with just a little green tea, grapefruit essential oil and non-alcoholic witch hazel, you can create a custom skincare product without even going out of your way. I love the way the aromas of the astringent green tea and fresh grapefruit come together. I hope you enjoy it as much as I do. Mornings have never felt so fresh.

METHOD

1. Add the boiling water and green tea bags to a ceramic or heatproof container (a glass jar works just fine) and steep for 10 minutes. Remove the tea bags and let the tea cool. I like to save the tea bags and put them in the fridge or freezer to use as cool eye compresses after a long day. It's important to let the tea cool fully because if you add essential oils to warm water, the volatile oils will evaporate and you won't get their full benefits.
2. Pour the green tea water into a mist bottle or glass jar with a lid.
3. Add the witch hazel and grapefruit essential oil to the tea. Shake well.

APPLICATION

1. Shake the toner vigorously before using it to evenly distribute the grapefruit essential oil throughout the liquid. It's normal for the oil to separate to the top of the mixture because the toner is completely natural and doesn't contain any toxic emulsifiers or additives.
2. After cleansing the face, mist the toner directly onto 2 cotton face pads. If you're keeping it in a jar, lightly dip the cotton face pads into the liquid.
3. With a damp cotton face pad in each hand, start in the middle of your face and make light downward and outward strokes from the middle of the nose out, from the middle of the forehead out and from the middle of the chin out.
4. Mist the toner directly onto a clean cotton face pad. Using the damp cotton face pad, start at the base of your neck and make light upward strokes toward the jawline.
5. Let the face toner sink into the skin for 10 to 15 seconds, then continue your facial routine. Follow with serum, moisturizer and/or eye creams.

Fennel and Lemongrass Face Toner (Combination Skin)

A nourishing toner that's gentle and dynamic enough for combination skin.

TIME: 30 minutes

MAKES: 8.8 ounces (264 mL) toner

YOU'LL NEED: a 12-ounce (360 mL) mist bottle or glass jar with lid and 3 organic cotton face pads

COMPONENTS

1 cup filtered water

2 teaspoons organic fennel seeds

1 tablespoon non-alcoholic witch hazel

4 drops lemongrass essential oil

STORAGE

Keep in the fridge for up to 2 weeks.

I love using this toner after a quick morning facial steam because it helps remove any other buildup or dirt released from my pores during the steam. It's also a great way to close the pores before applying makeup.

A facial toner should be simple and gentle, without any harsh drying agents. This helps maintain the skin's natural pH balance and won't prompt the skin to overproduce oil to compensate for the drying agents in the facial toner. Using botanicals and seeds helps create a new depth of aroma and properties in skincare. In this toner, I use fennel because it's known for being balancing and soothing for the stomach. This toner does the same for the skin, ensuring that it's calm and balanced yet energized and fresh. The lemongrass, much like fennel, is great at soothing and balancing and is also used as a digestive aid in cooking. Lemongrass essential oil also has gentle astringent properties, which makes it great for any oily areas in combination skin.

METHOD

1. In a small pot, add the filtered water and fennel seeds and bring to a boil. Keep at a boil for 5 minutes.
2. Remove from heat and allow the mixture to cool. Strain and discard the fennel seeds. It's important to let the mixture cool fully because if you add essential oils to warm water, the volatile oils will evaporate and you won't get their full benefits.
3. Pour the fennel liquid into a glass mist bottle or a glass jar with a lid.
4. Add the witch hazel and lemongrass essential oil to the mixture and shake well.

APPLICATION

1. Shake the toner vigorously before using it to evenly distribute the lemongrass essential oil throughout the liquid. It's normal for the oil to separate to the top of the mixture because the toner is completely natural and doesn't contain any toxic emulsifiers or additives.
2. After cleansing the face, mist the toner directly onto 2 cotton face pads.
3. With a damp cotton face pad in each hand, start in the middle of your face and make light downward and outward strokes from the middle of the nose out, from the middle of the forehead out and from the middle of the chin out.
4. Mist the toner directly onto a clean cotton face pad. Using the damp cotton face pad, start at the base of your neck and make light upward strokes toward the jawline.
5. Let the face toner sink into the skin for 10 to 15 seconds, then continue your facial routine. Follow with serum, moisturizer and/or eye creams.

Rosemary and Cedarwood Face Toner (Mature Skin)

A grounding toner for when you are craving the serenity of a hike in the woods.

TIME: 30 minutes

MAKES: 8 ounces (240 mL) toner

YOU'LL NEED: a 16-ounce (480 mL) mason jar or jar with a lid, an 8-ounce (240 mL) mist bottle and 3 organic cotton face pads

COMPONENTS

1 cup filtered water

2 sprigs fresh rosemary (or 2 sprigs dried rosemary)

1 teaspoon non-alcoholic witch hazel

3 drops cedarwood essential oil

There is something very comforting about this toner. Its simplicity and woodsy aroma make it more luxurious than other more citrus-centric aromas. I love the process of making this toner and enjoy using it during the winter months when my skin and nose are less excited about citrus and are craving some warm, woodsy scents. The rosemary helps with circulation and bringing blood flow to the surface of the skin, which can help with cell turn-over and regeneration. The cedarwood essential oil has slightly astringent properties, which can help tone and tighten the skin, and provides a deeply grounding aroma. It truly reminds me of waking up in a cabin in the woods, which helps me start my morning feeling calm and relaxed.

METHOD

1. Add the filtered water to a glass jar, then add the rosemary to the water so that the sprigs are completely covered. Close the lid of the jar and allow the mixture to sit in the fridge for 24 hours.
2. Strain and discard the rosemary. Add the witch hazel and cedarwood essential oil to the mixture. Pour the mixture into a mist bottle or keep it in the glass jar.

APPLICATION

1. Shake the toner vigorously before using it to evenly distribute the cedar-wood essential oil throughout the liquid. It's normal for the oil to separate to the top of the mixture because the toner is completely natural and doesn't contain any toxic emulsifiers or additives.
2. After cleansing the face, mist the toner directly onto 2 cotton face pads. If you're keeping it in a jar, lightly dip the cotton face pads into the liquid.
3. With a damp cotton face pad in each hand, start in the middle of your face and make light downward and outward strokes from the middle of the nose out, from the middle of the forehead out and from the middle of the chin out.
4. Mist the toner directly onto a clean cotton face pad. Using the damp cotton face pad, start at the base of your neck and make light upward strokes toward the jawline.
5. Let the face toner sink into the skin for 10 to 15 seconds, then continue your facial routine. Follow with serum, moisturizer and/or eye creams.

STORAGE

Keep in the fridge for up to 2 weeks.

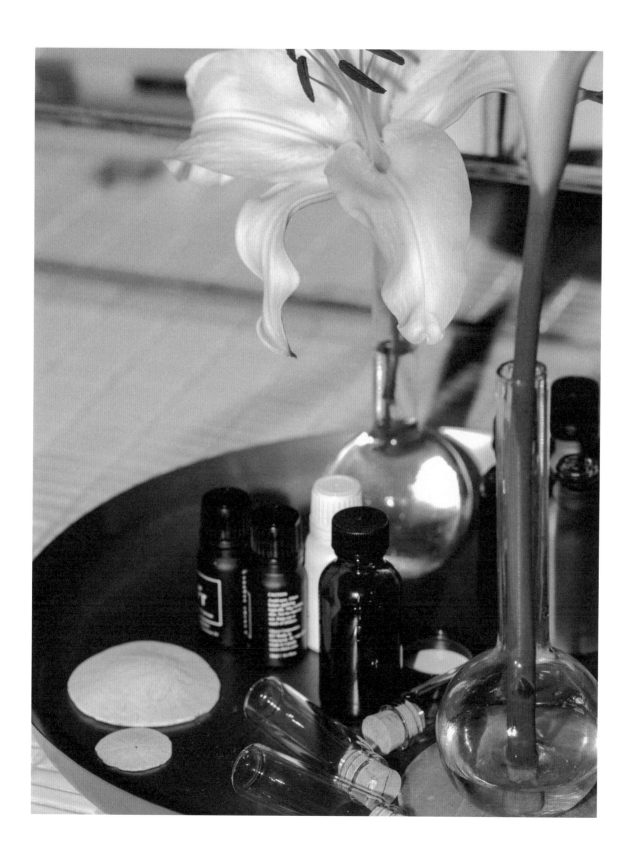

EASY EYE SERUMS

We live in a time when multi-tasking is glorified. Your success is measured by your degree of productivity: writing papers; holding down a job; nurturing relationships; answering calls, texts and emails promptly; updating your social media as well as perhaps owning your own side business or keeping up with your hobbies. Just thinking about it can be tiring. More on your plate equals less sleep. Less sleep means you are probably feeling and looking tired.

My life really changed when I realized the power and benefit of a good eye serum. Now, I really can't imagine my routine without it. In the past, those super-heavy, thick and expensive eye creams (you know, the ones your mother and grandmother used?) were a thing. Now, you can achieve the same results with much simpler recipes. These basic eye serums can be customized in a variety of ways to get the results you need at any given moment.

Serums are a great addition to a skincare routine because they penetrate more deeply into the skin than a traditional moisturizer. They're designed to mimic the skin's natural oils, which allows them to sink into the skin more easily. Serums are especially important around the eye area because the skin is more sensitive and thinner, so serums are incredibly effective in this area. In addition, the skin around your eyes and lips are often the first to show signs of aging—this is why I like to apply an eye serum daily and then apply anything left over to my upper lip area, right along the cupid's bow.

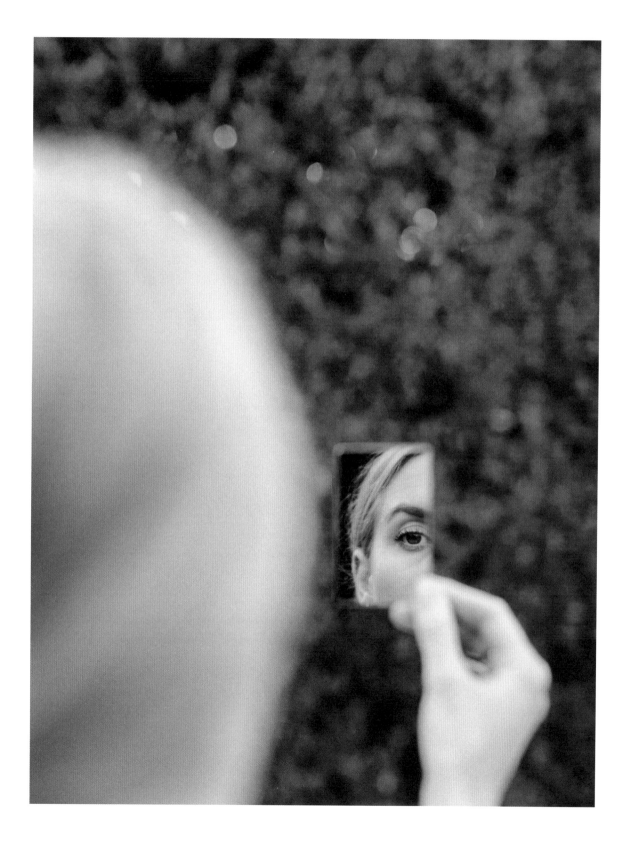

No-Snooze Eye Serum

An eye serum for when pressing snooze is not an option.

TIME: 2 minutes

MAKES: 0.17 ounce (5 mL) serum

YOU'LL NEED: a 0.3-ounce (10 mL) dropper bottle

COMPONENTS

1 teaspoon jojoba oil or base oil for your skin type (see page 29)

1 drop grapefruit essential oil

1 drop frankincense essential oil

1 vitamin E capsule

In my daily rituals, the time I feel most like I'm taking care of myself is when I apply an eye serum. The correct serum applied in the correct way takes your daily beauty ritual to another level and has become the favourite part of my beauty routine. Eye serums are very easy to make in small batches and to create on an ongoing basis. Hormones, stress, the climate and the hours of sleep we have each evening can have such an intense effect on our skin, and the area around our eyes is usually the first to show it.

The oils used in this recipe are great for moisturizing your skin and sinking into the thinner skin around the eye. Jojoba is used as the carrier oil for this recipe because it mimics the natural oil of the skin and helps carry the essential oils further into the dermis, making this serum perfect for mornings when you're running on less than 8 hours of sleep.

METHOD

1. Mix together all components in a dropper bottle.

APPLICATION

1. Using your fingers, lightly apply 2 to 3 drops of serum below your eyes. Starting at the outer edges of the brows, trace your fingers under the eyes and along the tops of the cheekbones toward the nose, ending just below the tear ducts. Repeat 2 to 3 times or until the serum is fully absorbed into the skin, about 1 to 2 minutes.

STORAGE

Keep at room temperature for up to 1 week or in the fridge for up to 1 month.

Gentle Warrior Eye Serum

An eye serum for tough mornings (Monday, I'm looking at you).

TIME: 2 minutes

MAKES: 0.3 ounce (10 mL) serum

YOU'LL NEED: a 0.3-ounce (10 mL) dropper bottle

COMPONENTS

1 teaspoon jojoba oil

1 teaspoon pomegranate seed oil

2 drops cedarwood essential oil

2 drops lavender essential oil

There are some days when you wake up and you know that the world is going to come at you. I use this serum on those mornings—the ones when you feel like you need a little layer to protect you. Carving out that extra minute in my morning routine to apply this serum correctly helps me start the day feeling just a little more centred. The lavender essential oil is incredibly relaxing, while the cedarwood is grounding—both work together to make me feel like I can take on anything the day throws at me.

METHOD

1. Mix together all components in a dropper bottle.

APPLICATION

1. Using your fingers, lightly apply 2 to 3 drops of serum below your eyes. Starting at the outer edges of the brows, trace your fingers under the eyes and along the tops of the cheekbones toward the nose, ending just below the tear ducts. Repeat 2 to 3 times or until the serum is fully absorbed into the skin, about 1 to 2 minutes.

STORAGE

Keep at room temperature for up to 1 week or in the fridge for up to 1 month.

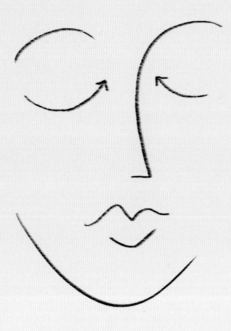

HOW TO APPLY EYE SERUM: LYMPHATIC DRAINAGE MASSAGE TECHNIQUE

Eye serum is traditionally applied to the eye area (scientifically known as the orbital area) by applying a drop and massaging it into the area surrounding the eye. While this technique is readily used today in facials and for applying makeup, another method of applying serum takes into account the way lymph naturally drains from the face. This method is known as a lymphatic drainage massage and can help reduce puffiness and fluid retention while also helping the serum absorb even deeper into the skin.

STEPS

1. Apply 1 drop of serum to the tips of your fingers and lightly press into the thin skin under the eye, starting at the outer corner and moving to the inner corner.
2. Apply 1 drop of serum to each ring finger and press the fingers into the inner corners of the eye on the bridge of the nose between the two eyes.
3. Close your eyes and breathe deeply.
4. Apply 1 more drop of serum to each ring finger and press lightly into the middle of the brow bone. Trace the finger from the upper inner corner of the brow along the brow to the outer corner.

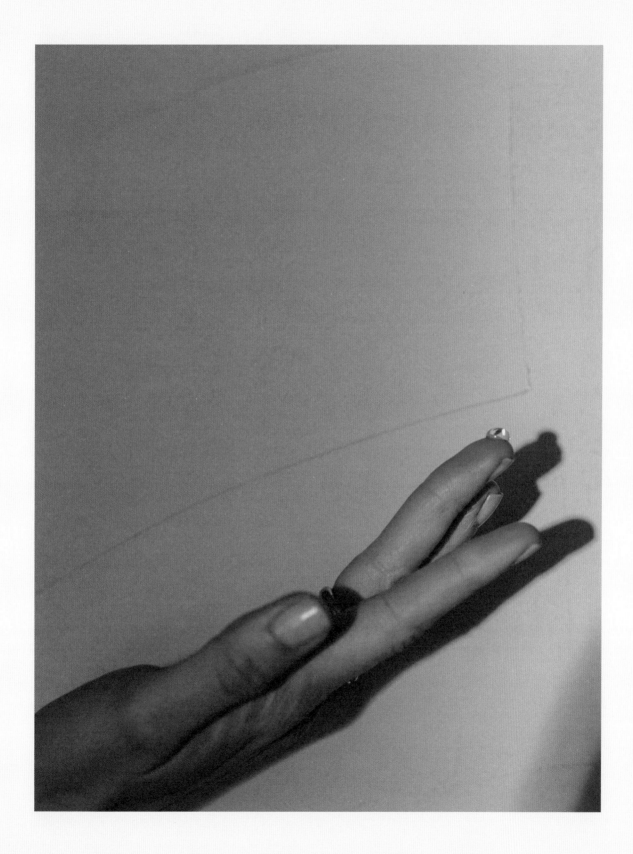

HOMEMADE HAIR OILS

It took a little convincing for me to try using a hair oil in my morning routine. Because I have straight and fine hair, I was worried it would get greasy or weighed down. After finally trying a few, I quickly realized that either the hair oils I was experimenting with contained the wrong ingredients or I was applying them in the wrong way. Brushing your hair and applying hair oil in the correct way can make all the difference.

Creating a custom hair oil can be helpful for any hair type—oily, dry, curly or pin straight. After colouring my hair and finally returning to my natural colour, I knew I had to incorporate a daily ritual that added a little moisture back into my hair. I started mixing my own hair oil and applying it to the ends of my hair after curling it in the mornings. I've noticed that it has helped with damage created by heat, as well as with fly-away hair during drier temperatures.

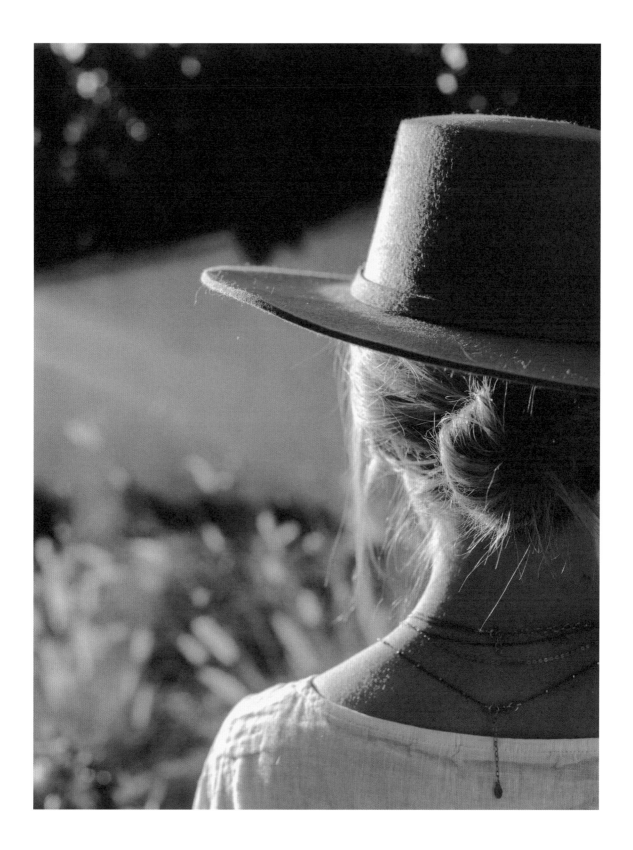

Everyday Hair Oil

A hair oil that defies any notions of greasy.

TIME: 2 minutes
MAKES: 0.85 ounce (25 mL)
hair oil
YOU'LL NEED: a 1-ounce
(30 mL) dropper bottle

COMPONENTS

5 teaspoons base oil of your
choice (see page 29)

8 drops lavender essential oil

5 drops rosemary essential oil

This hair oil is my favourite way to end a shower or bath, and I usually apply a few drops after I've applied heat stress to my hair or scalp, to help replace moisture that may have been lost. This is a great everyday oil that isn't too heavy and is good for all seasons. In this recipe, I include lavender essential oil because it helps keep hair shafts and follicles clear of bacteria, giving your hair a chance to breathe. It's also known for its ability to soothe your scalp (and your mind) courtesy of its natural sedative properties. Rosemary essential oil is a staple when it comes to custom hair products, as it helps improve cellular metabolism, which stimulates hair growth by keeping the follicles active. It also gives you this tingly feeling, which I love. Sometimes I add a little cedarwood essential oil if I'm using the hair oil in the evenings because it adds a cozy depth to the aroma. I like using grapeseed oil as a base oil because it is really light and nice for daily use.

METHOD
1. Mix together all components in a dropper bottle.

APPLICATION
1. Apply a few drops of the hair oil to the ends of wet or dry hair. For wet hair, use 1 teaspoon. For dry hair, I put just 1 drop in the palm of my hand, then use my fingers to lightly smooth it through the ends of my hair, making sure it's distributed evenly.

STORAGE
Keep in a cool, dry place away from direct sunlight or severe temperature changes for up to 1 month.

Rosemary Brow Salve

A nourishing salve for great morning brows that stay in place all day.

TIME: 15 minutes

MAKES: 1.86 ounces (55 mL) brow salve

YOU'LL NEED: 2 double boilers and a 2-ounce (60 mL) container with a lid

COMPONENTS

4 teaspoons shea butter

1 tablespoon jojoba oil

1 teaspoon rosehip oil

1 tablespoon beeswax (I like natural organic beeswax pellets)

5 drops rosemary essential oil

2 drops lemon essential oil

1 drop geranium essential oil

Brows definitely have had a renaissance moment. Gone are the days when *thin* was in. Now, it's all about bold, healthy brows, and that's something I can easily get behind. I apply this brow salve in the morning and, thanks to the semi-solid state of the shea butter and beeswax, it helps lock in moisture and keep my brows in place all day.

On top of being ultra-moisturizing, the shea butter helps house all the benefits of the essential oils. In this recipe, I use rosehip oil because it's super nourishing, while rosemary essential oil is refreshing and rejuvenating to the hair follicles and helps promote full, healthy brows. Geranium essential oil has a natural, slightly minty aroma that I absolutely love, and it leaves the brows tingling a bit, which promotes healthy hair follicles.

METHOD

1. Using a double boiler, warm the shea butter over low heat. As it melts, add the jojoba oil and rosehip oil. Stir the mixture, being careful to keep the temperature low so that you don't overheat the oils. Leave the double boiler on low heat so that the mixture doesn't start to cool and solidify.
2. Using another double boiler, heat the beeswax over low, gentle heat until it melts—again, making sure not to boil the wax or let it get it too hot.
3. When the shea butter mixture and the beeswax are completely melted, add the beeswax slowly to the shea butter mixture. Stir to combine.
4. Remove from the heat and continue to stir until the mixture starts to cool, turning a milky colour and achieving a thicker texture. As the mixture cools, add all essential oils while stirring continuously.
5. While the mixture is still liquid, pour it into the container and let sit uncovered to cool.

APPLICATION

1. Warm the salve in your fingertips, then apply a pea-sized amount to your brows as part of your morning routine or as a fresh pick-me-up throughout the day.

STORAGE

Keep in a cool, dry place away from direct sunlight or severe temperature changes for up to 3 months.

MORNING FACE MASKS

Masks and exfoliating face scrubs can be lengthy, time-consuming processes that are often associated with Friday night candlelit baths and wine (a scenario most of us aren't privy to on a regular basis). But the benefits and invigorating experience of a mask and exfoliation shouldn't be lost on those of us with busy schedules. So, in keeping with our goal of elevating the simple and very normal parts of your day, I designed these invigorating and exfoliating facial masks to fit into your existing morning ritual. The great thing about these recipes is that you can blend the mask in a ceramic bowl or in a mason jar with a lid and keep them in your shower for up to 1 week. Who doesn't love an easy spa experience that no one else in your home will know you're having? Secret spa time is my favourite spa time.

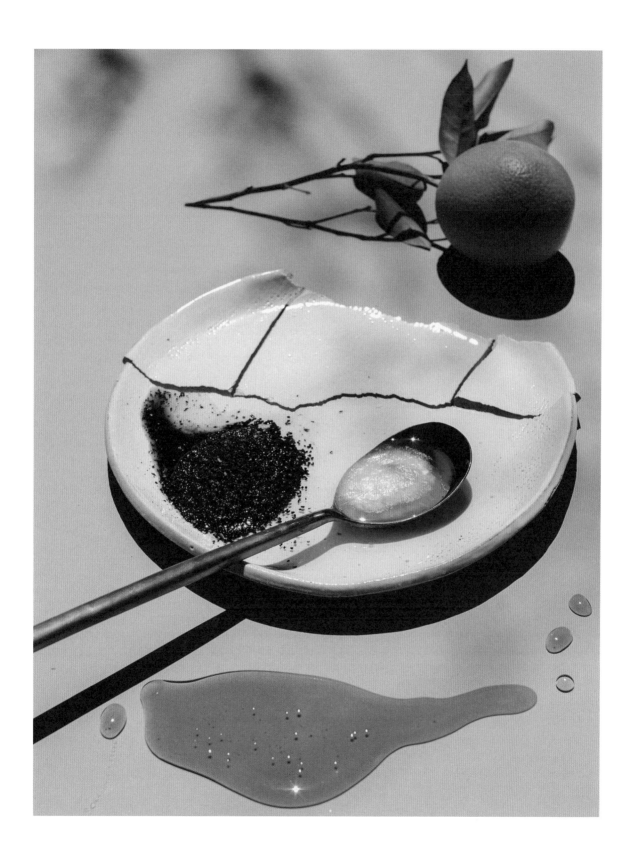

Coconut Coffee Orange Honey Face Mask

An invigorating face mask that takes your morning shower to another level.

TIME: 5 minutes

MAKES: 3.38 ounces (100 mL) of face mask

YOU'LL NEED: a small bowl or glass jar

COMPONENTS

2 tablespoons organic solid virgin coconut oil

2 teaspoons organic liquid honey

6 drops sweet orange essential oil

4 tablespoons organic coffee grounds

The components of this face mask were chosen for both their aromas and their benefits to the skin. Coconut oil has natural antimicrobial properties and helps soothe and moisturize the skin, while coffee is super simulating to the skin. If coffee wasn't already one of your favourite things in the world, it is now. Not only does it increase circulation and blood flow to the dermis, but it also exfoliates the skin in a gentle way and adds a smooth finish. Honey is great for nourishing and balancing the complexion, as well as for helping your skin absorb and retain moisture. Whenever I use this mask, it helps keep my skin soft, dewy and glowing. Honey also has natural antibacterial and antimicrobial properties, which makes it a great option for when an unexpected blemish pops up.

The takeaway for this recipe is that it's a simple way to sneak a spa moment into your boring morning shower routine. The best part? There's zero mess involved because it all takes place in the shower.

METHOD

1. Add the coconut oil, honey and sweet orange essential oil to a small bowl or glass jar.
2. Mix the coffee grounds into the oil and honey mixture until combined.

APPLICATION

1. Moisten the face with warm shower water to help open the pores and soften the skin.
2. Put 2 to 3 teaspoons of the face mask mixture on your fingertips and massage it onto your face in small circular upward motions, avoiding the eyes.
3. Leave the mask on your face while you finish your morning shower routine—shampooing, conditioning, washing your body. Allow the mask to sit for at least 5 minutes before rinsing it off with warm shower water.

STORAGE

Keep the face mask in a covered bowl or jar with a lid in the shower for up to 1 week. Try to prevent water from getting into the bowl or jar to ensure that it lasts the full week. You can also keep it in the fridge for up to 2 weeks.

Sweet and Soothing Oats and Honey Face Mask

A nourishing face mask you'll wish you could eat.

TIME: 5 minutes

MAKES: 2.36 ounces (70 mL) face mask

YOU'LL NEED: a small bowl or glass jar

COMPONENTS

2 tablespoons sweet almond oil

2 teaspoons organic liquid honey

2 drops geranium essential oil

2 tablespoons quick oats

This is one of my favourite morning rituals, especially on days I know will be intense and when a lot will be coming at me. I love the gentle aroma and feeing of oatmeal, especially in the winter when my skin is a little more dry and sensitive. On days when you don't have time to make oatmeal in the morning, the aroma and gentle experience of this shower mask makes up for that and adds a cozy and gentle energy to the morning hustle. It's a welcomed experience in my morning routine before the world comes at me.

METHOD

1. Add the sweet almond oil, honey and geranium essential oil to a small bowl or glass jar.
2. Add the quick oats and stir into the oil and honey mixture.

APPLICATION

1. Moisten the face with warm shower water to help open the pores and soften the skin.
2. Put 2 to 3 teaspoons of the face mask mixture on your fingertips and massage it onto your face in small circular upward motions, avoiding the eyes.
3. Leave the mask on your face while you finish your morning shower routine— shampooing, conditioning, washing your body. Allow the mask to sit for at least 5 minutes before rinsing it off with warm shower water.

STORAGE

Keep the face mask in a covered bowl or jar with a lid in the shower for up to 1 week. Try to prevent water from getting into the bowl or jar to ensure that it lasts the full week. You can also keep it in the fridge for up to 2 weeks.

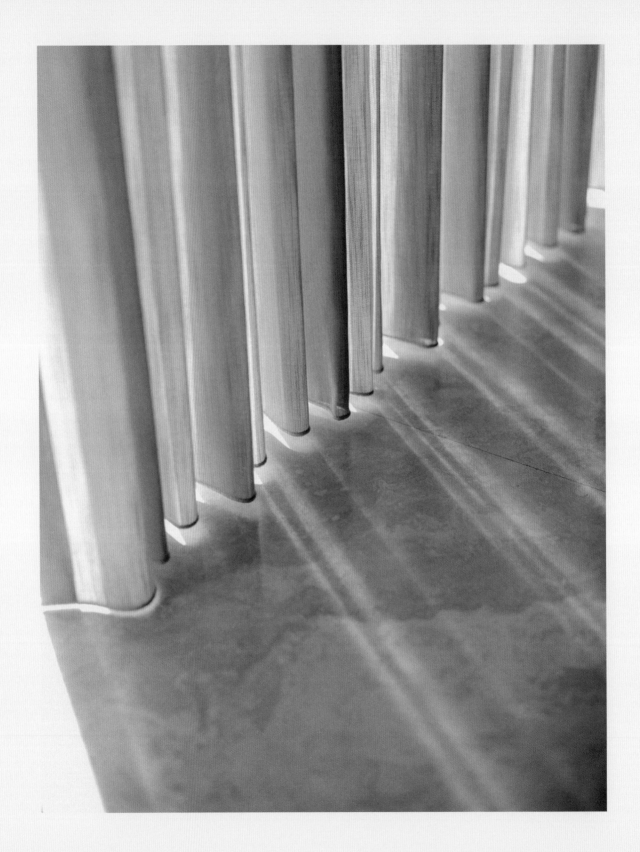

MAKING YOURSELF A MORNING PERSON

Some people are naturally more "morning people" than others, but there are simple ways to trigger the brain and body into waking up that are more natural than hitting snooze and reaching for an espresso (although I'm no stranger to doing both). As someone who is a morning person but also puts in late hours during the workweek, I've created some very strategic practices through trial and error (and research) that help me wake up and feel more refreshed by the time I get to the office.

In keeping with the theme of this book, these are incredibly simple tips that shouldn't change your current routine too much. They're really just ways to improve your daily morning habits and make them work a little more in your favour; this way, they become less of a necessity and more of an elevating experience for your wellness.

DRINK WATER

Many wellness publications and books talk about drinking warm lemon water in the morning. Regardless of whether the water has lemon in it, drinking room-temperature (or warm) water in the morning is an incredibly effective way to start your day. After learning about the benefits of water in the morning, I realized that it actually has significant positive effects on your brain, your metabolism and your skin (a few things I care tremendously about). Your body is slightly dehydrated in the morning from breathing for 8 hours, not taking in liquids and possibly sweating. So, when you start the day off with a sugary breakfast and a dehydrating coffee, you can bet you're only going to crash and get a headache an hour later, after becoming even more dehydrated. So, for the sake of my brain (and skin), I decided that if there was one wellness practice I would take seriously, it would be hydration.

So, how to remember and how much to drink? I bought myself a glass carafe that I keep beside my bed with exactly 4 cups of water in it. I fill it up and put it beside my bed each night—it has a little glass that covers it, which makes for a stylish and convenient drinking experience. When I wake up, the first thing I do after turning off my alarm (and saying good morning to my dog beside me) is reach for the carafe of water. I don't drink the whole thing while still in bed, but I try to get through at least half of it; then I finish the other half while putting on my makeup and waiting for my coffee to brew. This way, if I've done nothing else for my wellness that day, I know I've started the day rehydrated.

SET THE AROMA

A diffuser in the morning can change the way you wake up. I keep one by my bed and use a relaxing blend in the evening and a citrus blend in the morning.

Keep a diffuser in your kitchen, bedroom or bathroom and diffuse oils that naturally help you wake up. I love diffusing sweet orange and peppermint essential oils in the morning in the spring and summer months. In the fall, I usually go for something a bit more woodsy, such as spruce essential oil, and pair it with grapefruit essential oil.

Another simple idea for the morning is to bring eucalyptus essential oil into the shower. For an easy eucalyptus steam spa experience, simply add 2 to 5 drops of eucalyptus essential oil to your palms and rub your hands briskly together. Hold your palms up and allow the warmth of the steam to help the volatile oils in the essential oil release into the air. Take three deep breaths and focus on filling up your lungs with energizing oxygen.

STRETCH IN BED

There are hundreds of morning yoga routines on the internet and a million books about how to design and create the perfect morning yoga practice. In complete and total honesty, mornings are some of my most productive hours, and by the time I'm awake, my brain is already working really fast. That said, the last thing I want to do is an ultra-meditative yoga practice. What I've designed instead is a simple morning stretch I call "Feet in the Air" to promote circulation and move blood flow throughout the brain and body. To practise this stretch, lay on your back in bed, put your legs and feet in the air and gently pedal your feet back and forth. Repeat for 1 to 2 minutes. This helps get blood to the brain and naturally helps you feel alert and energized.

CREATE A HEALTHIER COFFEE RITUAL

There is a lot of talk about healthier coffee alternatives and ways to make the buzz and energy of caffeine interact with your metabolism in a more balanced way. This was especially interesting to me because I'm not a big breakfast eater (but I love coffee) and would usually opt for a great cappuccino and a bite-sized something over a super-filling breakfast. With experimentation, I've learned to adapt my morning coffee into a healthier experience that leaves me feeling physically and mentally nourished—so that by the time I get to the office, my energy is more balanced.

BALANCED BREW

INGREDIENTS

1 cup brewed organic coffee (I make mine in a French press)

1 to 2 teaspoons organic solid virgin coconut oil

4 tablespoons organic unsweetened coconut or cashew milk (homemade if you have time)

¼ teaspoon organic pure vanilla extract

½ teaspoon organic maca root powder

Pinch of cinnamon

½ teaspoon organic liquid honey or organic maple syrup

Add all ingredients to your favourite mug and stir to combine. For a more luxurious experience, add the ingredients to a blender and mix on high speed for 10 seconds until the mixture becomes foamy and frothy. Pour in a mug and enjoy.

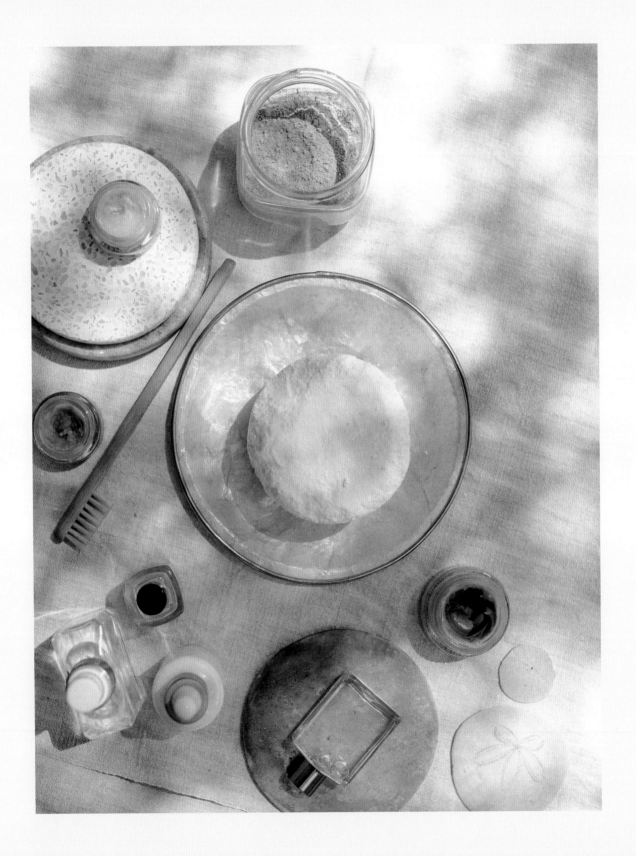

AFTERNOON BEAUTY RITUALS

In the afternoon, I'm usually running between meetings, on calls, or doing errands on the weekend and prepping for travel. My wellness and beauty practices are the last thing on my mind, but hectic afternoons are surprisingly some of the easiest times to sneak in new beauty rituals. Since most of our afternoons during the week are quite scheduled, it makes carving out specific times to try new practices pretty doable. Put it in your calendar and you're good to go (kidding . . . only sort of).

I've created these rituals and recipes to fit seamlessly into the places you may be in the afternoon: your desk, the boardroom, on the subway, in your living room. The goal for these recipes is to make it easy for you to take some time for yourself when you need it most.

It's interesting when you start experimenting with self-care routines throughout your day. Remembering to take a few deep breaths is often more beneficial than consuming more caffeine and a stretch at your desk can fill the lungs and get the blood going in a way that a sugary snack at 3 pm can't.

Regaining your stamina, energy and motivation during the middle of the day can help push you over the finish line in a productive and inspiring way, leaving you at 5 pm with more perspective and energy than if you had "powered through" your day by forgetting to drink water, breathe, stretch and carve out even just 30 seconds for yourself.

The world needs you to take care of yourself so you can be your best self, and that's especially important in the afternoon amid all the hustle.

Natural Lip Balms

A basic balm recipe for keeping lips plump and hydrated

TIME: 5 minutes

MAKES: 0.85 ounce (25 mL) lip balm

YOU'LL NEED: a double boiler, a spoon and a 1-ounce (30 mL) tin or glass container with a lid

COMPONENTS

2 teaspoons organic solid virgin coconut oil

2 teaspoons organic cocoa butter

1 teaspoon organic beeswax

5 drops essential oils based on seasonal blends (see page 77)

½ teaspoon organic beet root powder (optional, for tinting)

Lip balms are a super-easy and fun way to introduce non-toxic natural beauty products into your routine. This lip balm is made for any time of day and can be customized for the season so that your everyday essential incorporates different aromas at each time of the year. Plus, it takes only 5 minutes to make, so you could make lip balms for your car, your purse and your desk in 15 minutes flat.

To live simply and naturally, one of the easiest green beauty products you can switch to is homemade, natural lip balm. With it being so close to my lips, I love knowing that I've made the product I'm using and that it's as natural and nourishing as possible.

METHOD

1. In a double boiler over low heat, combine the coconut oil, cocoa butter and beeswax and stir until melted.
2. Remove from heat and continue stirring. When the mixture begins to cool, it will begin to thicken and the colour will turn milky; at this time, add the essential oils and beet powder (if using) and continue stirring.
3. Pour the mixture into the container and let cool without a lid (covering it results in condensation, which prevents the balm from drying correctly). Allow the balm to cool for 6 to 8 hours (or overnight), then cover.

APPLICATION

1. Using your fingers, apply the natural lip balm to your lips as desired throughout the day.

STORAGE

Keep in a cool, dry place (or your purse) for up to 3 months.

Seasonal Essential Oil Lip Balm Blends

Each of the following essential oil blends is designed to create a seasonal twist on an everyday essential.

SPRING FLORAL NATURAL LIP BALM
Feminine and floral, like an exotic bouquet.
3 drops geranium essential oil
2 drops ylang ylang essential oil

SUMMER CITRUS NATURAL LIP BALM
Warm and inviting, like a citrus grove on a warm day.
2 drops bergamot essential oil
2 drops grapefruit essential oil
1 drop lemongrass essential oil

FALL HERBAL NATURAL LIP BALM
Woodsy and crisp, like a dewy fall hike.
4 drops peppermint essential oil
1 drop cedarwood essential oil

WINTER FRESH TINTED NATURAL LIP BALM
Cooling and invigorating, like an icy breath of fresh air.
3 drops lemon essential oil
2 drops peppermint essential oil
1 teaspoon organic beet root powder

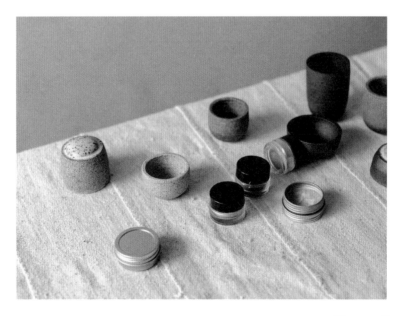

FACE MISTS FOR THE DAILY GRIND

Sometimes the days can get away from you—between meetings, projects, calls, family and friends, there are days when it might be hard to remember if you've showered. On other days, you may not have time to freshen up at home before heading out to a dinner, soccer practice or workout class. Regardless of your schedule, you can feel a little more prepared for whatever the day throws at you by incorporating each of these naturally toning face mists into different parts of your daily routine. The essential oils chosen are made specifically for elevating simple moments throughout your day.

These toning face mists are my favourite way to refresh and recharge through-out a busy day. Beyond their amazing smell, the simple inhalation of the facial mist reminds me to breathe deeply and reset.

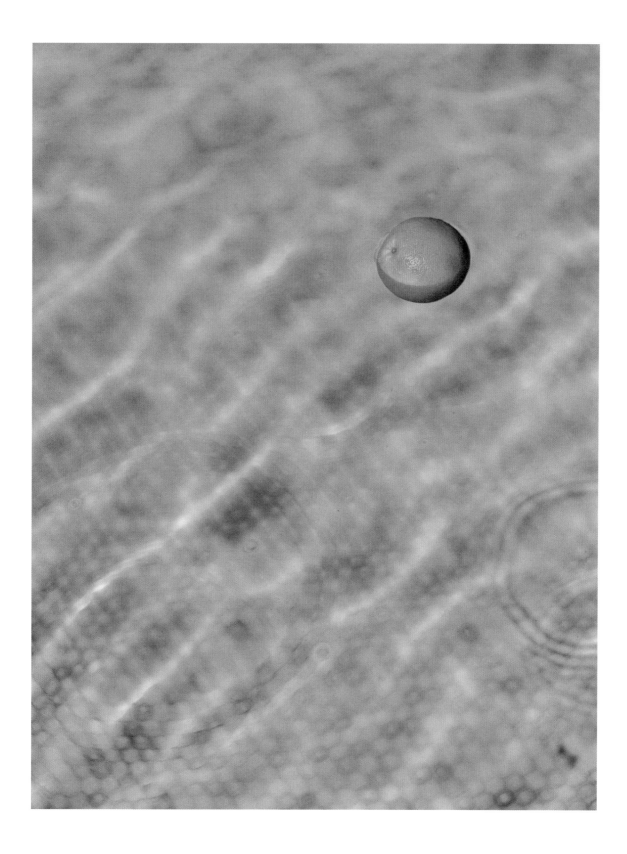

Energizing Face Mist

A rejuvenating midday mist for when you can't stop, won't stop.

TIME: 2 minutes

MAKES: 1 ounce (30 mL) face mist

YOU'LL NEED: a 1-ounce (30 mL) mist bottle

COMPONENTS

4 teaspoons filtered water

2 teaspoons non-alcoholic witch hazel

6 drops spruce essential oil

5 drops grapefruit essential oil

4 drops lemon essential oil

With a fresh citrus blend of natural cold-pressed oils, this energizing facial mist is a favourite to use both in the morning to set my makeup and in the afternoon around 3 pm to refresh myself in lieu of (or along with) another espresso.

METHOD

1. Combine all components in the mist bottle.
2. Shake well before each use.

APPLICATION

1. Mist face and/or body. Breathe deeply.

STORAGE

Keep in a cool, dark place for 2 to 3 months. Because there is water in the mist (and no preservatives), make sure to keep it away from direct sunlight.

Balancing Face Mist

A cleansing, refreshing mist for when you need to skip the shower.

TIME: 2 minutes

MAKES: 1 ounce (30 mL) face mist

YOU'LL NEED: a 1-ounce (30 mL) mist bottle

COMPONENTS

4 teaspoons filtered water

2 teaspoons non-alcoholic witch hazel

5 drops geranium essential oil

5 drops tea tree essential oil

This is my favourite toning facial mist. I use it on my face, neck and sometimes down my shirt or back in lieu of a shower before heading out to a dinner or event straight from work. This perfect mix of minty geranium essential oil and pungent tea tree essential oil quite literally smells like a fresh shower in a bottle. I love using this face mist at lunchtime, too, as a midday reset before I tackle the rest of my day (and night).

METHOD

1. Combine all components in the mist bottle.
2. Shake well before each use.

APPLICATION

1. Mist face and/or body. Breathe deeply.

STORAGE

Keep in a cool, dark place for 2 to 3 months. Because there is water in the mist (and no preservatives), make sure to keep it away from direct sunlight.

Calming Face Mist

A soothing mist that will leave you saying "ahhhhhhh."

TIME: 2 minutes

MAKES: 1 ounce (30 mL) face mist

YOU'LL NEED: a 1-ounce (30 mL) mist bottle

COMPONENTS

4 teaspoons filtered water

2 teaspoons non-alcoholic witch hazel

5 drops lavender essential oil

4 drops cedarwood essential oil

1 drop ylang ylang essential oil

When I want a naturally calming face toner that eases both my skin and my senses, I always grab these ingredients and whip up a batch of calming face mist. It's made with a completely natural blend of essential oils that helps promote deep breathing and has a grounding quality.

I've made this simple recipe on the fly in the past, before a presentation or a long red-eye flight, knowing that I'll be feeling some redness in my skin and some restlessness in my legs. The calming lavender and grounding cedarwood essential oils help make me feel like I'm in a spa, regardless of whether I'm about to walk into a boardroom or I'm 35,000 feet in the air. I hope this calming toner will give you as much respite as it has given me.

METHOD

1. Combine all components in the mist bottle.
2. Shake well before each use.

APPLICATION

1. Mist face and/or body. Breathe deeply.

STORAGE

Keep in a cool, dark place for 2 to 3 months. Because there is water in the mist (and no preservatives), make sure to keep it away from direct sunlight.

TEA TONERS FOR EVERYDAY REFRESHES

I've been a tea fan for many years, but it wasn't until recently that I discovered the topical benefits of my favourite teas. The benefits of green, black and herbal tea you get from consuming them are very similar to the ones you experience when they're applied topically to the skin. These tea toners are best made in small batches and kept in the fridge for ultimate freshness, while also increasing their cooling and refreshing properties. Here are my go-to recipes for each type of tea found most often in my kitchen. I prefer using organic teas, but there's no need to use anything fancy or special—a simple tea bag or loose leaf tea will do.

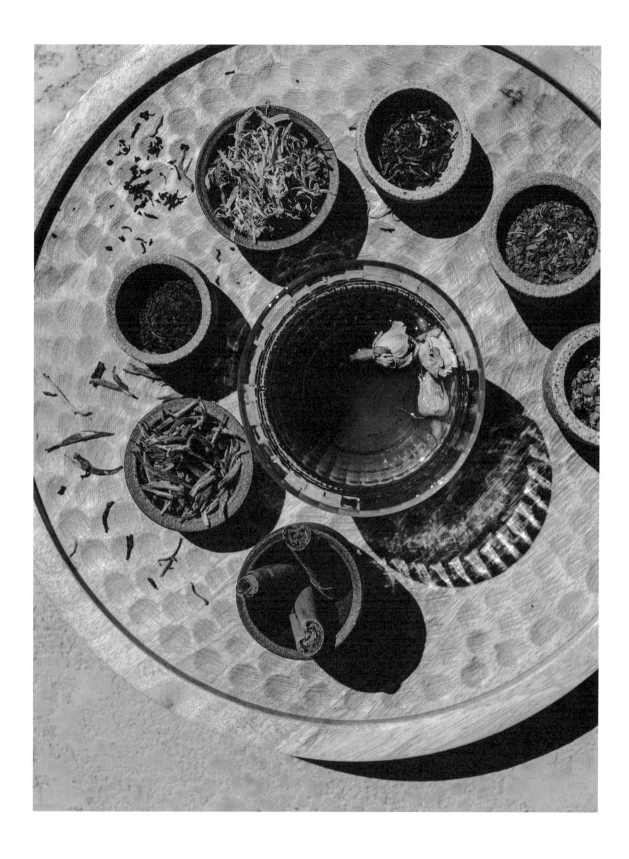

Green Tea Face Toner

A refreshing, feminine tea toner perfect for an afternoon reset.

TIME: 15 minutes

MAKES: 1 ounce (30 mL) tea toner

YOU'LL NEED: a 1-ounce (30 mL) mist bottle and 2 organic cotton face pads

COMPONENTS

1 cup boiling filtered water

1 teaspoon loose leaf organic green tea or 1 organic green tea bag

7 drops rosemary essential oil

7 drops geranium essential oil

Applying green tea to the skin is a beautiful and natural way to balance and tone your complexion. The antioxidants found in the tea can help naturally balance the skin's pH and have a slight mattifying effect—leaving the skin not too dry but not too oily. This green tea toner is my favourite weekend DIY project that turns a simple tea on a Saturday morning into a beauty product that will last through the week.

For best results, I love keeping this toner in the fridge, especially during warmer months, to ensure that it stays completely fresh and germ-free since it contains no preservatives. Regardless of how long you keep it, making more shouldn't be too much trouble—you can even make it daily if sipping green tea is part of your afternoon routine.

METHOD

1. Add the boiling water and loose leaf tea or tea bag to a cup and let steep for 10 minutes. Strain the tea leaves or remove the tea bag and set aside 2 tablespoons of steeped green tea to cool completely. It's important to let the tea cool fully because if you add essential oils to warm water, the volatile oils will evaporate and you won't get their full benefits. You can drink the leftover tea hot or cold as an afternoon refreshment.
2. Pour the reserved cold green tea into the mist bottle and add the essential oils.
3. Shake well before each use.

APPLICATION

1. Mist the green tea face toner onto 2 cotton face pads.
2. Using a cotton face pad in each hand, wipe from the centre of the face outward and downward.
3. Take 3 deep breaths.
4. Finish with your favourite face oil to complete your afternoon refresh beauty routine.

STORAGE

Keep in a cool, dark place for up to 2 weeks. I like to store my toner in the fridge, so that it feels extra refreshing on the skin.

Black Tea Face Toner

A mattifying tea toner to apply before that big presentation.

TIME: 15 minutes

MAKES: 1 ounce (30 mL) tea toner

YOU'LL NEED: a 1-ounce (30 mL) mist bottle and 2 organic cotton face pads

COMPONENTS

1 cup boiling filtered water

1 teaspoon loose leaf organic black tea or 1 organic black tea bag

7 drops lavender essential oil

7 drops frankincense essential oil

The most astringent of the teas, black tea is known for its tightening and slightly drying qualities, making it best suited for those with slightly more oily skin. It's also a great option if you live or are travelling somewhere humid. I love making this toner and using it in the afternoon when I have oily patches or before a meeting when my skin needs to be a little more matte naturally.

METHOD

1. Add the boiling water and loose leaf tea or tea bag to a cup and let steep for 10 minutes. Strain the tea leaves or remove the tea bag and set aside 2 tablespoons of steeped black tea to cool completely. It's important to let the tea cool fully because if you add essential oils to warm water, the volatile oils will evaporate and you won't get their full benefits. You can drink the leftover tea hot or cold as an afternoon refreshment.
2. Pour the reserved cold black tea into the mist bottle and add the essential oils.
3. Shake well before each use.

APPLICATION

1. Mist the black tea face toner onto 2 cotton face pads.
2. Using a cotton face pad in each hand, wipe from the centre of the face outward and downward.
3. Take 3 deep breaths.
4. Finish with your favourite face oil to complete your afternoon refresh beauty routine.

STORAGE

Keep in a cool, dark place for up to 2 weeks. I like to store my toner in the fridge, so that it feels extra refreshing on the skin.

Herbal Tea Face Toner

A soothing tea toner for after travel, tears or too much sun.

TIME: 15 minutes

MAKES: 1 ounce (30 mL) tea toner

YOU'LL NEED: a 1-ounce (30 mL) mist bottle and 2 organic cotton face pads

COMPONENTS

1 cup boiling filtered water

1 teaspoon loose leaf organic peppermint tea or 1 organic peppermint tea bag

7 drops lemongrass essential oil

7 drops grapefruit essential oil

A peppermint tea toner is something I reach for when I'm travelling because it can help decrease redness in the skin, and peppermint tea is easy to find in most hotel rooms. This toner is great to use in the afternoon after a flight or a long commute, or after you've spent a little too much time in the sun. Peppermint is great for decreasing redness and swelling—I've also been known to use this toner after a good cry to help decrease the resulting redness and puffiness.

METHOD

1. Add the boiling water and loose leaf tea or tea bag to a cup and let steep for 10 minutes. Strain the tea leaves or remove the tea bag and set aside 2 tablespoons of steeped peppermint tea to cool completely. It's important to let the tea cool fully because if you add essential oils to warm water, the volatile oils will evaporate and you won't get their full benefits. You can drink the leftover tea hot or cold as an afternoon refreshment.
2. Pour the reserved cold peppermint tea into the mist bottle and add the essential oils.
3. Shake well before each use.

APPLICATION

1. Mist the peppermint tea face toner onto 2 cotton face pads.
2. Using a cotton face pad in each hand, wipe from the centre of the face outward and downward.
3. Take 3 deep breaths.
4. Finish with your favourite face oil to complete your afternoon refresh beauty routine.

STORAGE

Keep in a cool, dark place for up to 2 weeks. I like to store my toner in the fridge, so that it feels extra refreshing on the skin.

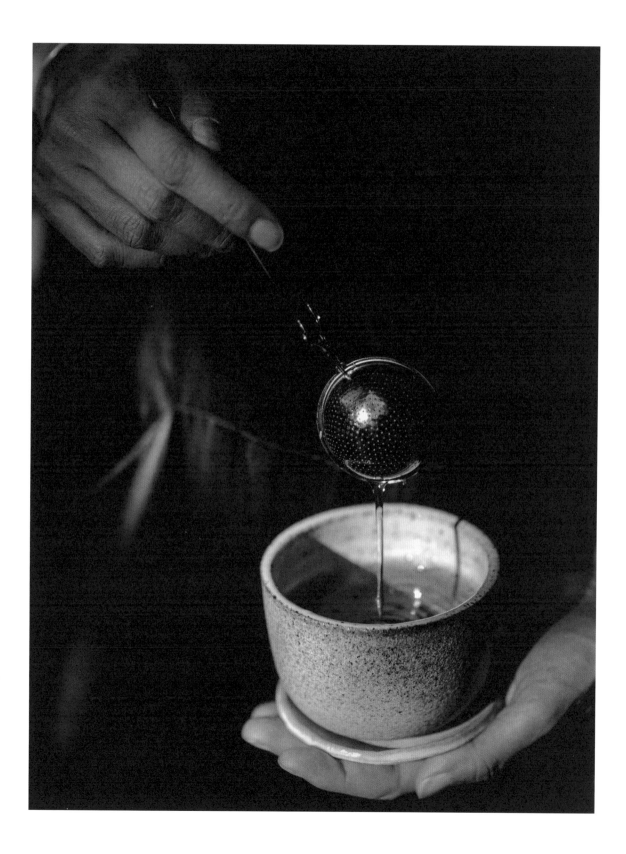

Moisturizing Blemish Spot Treatment

A blemish spot treatment you can actually apply at your desk.

TIME: 3 minutes

MAKES: 0.5 ounce (15 mL) spot treatment

YOU'LL NEED: a 0.5-ounce (15 mL) dropper bottle

COMPONENTS

BASE OILS
2 teaspoons unrefined organic avocado oil

¾ teaspoon jojoba oil

COMPLEX OIL
½ teaspoon raspberry seed oil

ESSENTIAL OILS
10 drops tea tree essential oil

8 drops lemon essential oil

8 drops geranium essential oil

This moisturizing blemish spot treatment is always in my bag. It's an ultra-hydrating oil that sinks into the skin and can be applied throughout the day—especially in the afternoon when oil production is high.

A dynamic and effective blemish treatment should do two things: moisturize and decrease the oil and bacteria in the area. Most store-bought treatments focus on the drying aspect. This blend is different; it takes a more holistic approach to blemish-prone skin by using hydrating base oils and balancing complex oils and essential oils that help decrease bacteria, control oil and tone and balance the skin.

Avocado and jojoba are the two base oils that most mimic the consistency of oil naturally found in the skin. This means they sink into the skin instead of adding a shiny layer on its surface (not something you want at 1 pm). Raspberry seed oil is full of vitamin E, which makes it a powerful antioxidant and helps decrease redness. Raspberry seed oil also has reportedly very high levels of phytosterols, which help reduce water loss throughout the skin layers—thus keeping skin moisturized and more hydrated instead of firm and tight. Beyond hydration, phytosterols have also been shown to help promote the natural cycle of skin repair and regeneration after damage from environmental factors, such as sun damage.

METHOD
1. Combine the base oils, complex oil and essential oils in a dropper bottle.
2. Put the cap on the dropper bottle and shake well.

APPLICATION
1. Using a clean finger or cotton swab, apply 1 drop of spot treatment directly on a blemish. For more preventative application, apply 1 drop to any place you're worried a blemish might pop up (like your T-zone, chin or cheeks) and rub into the skin, avoiding the eyes.

STORAGE
Keep in a cool, dry place away from direct sunlight (or in your purse for everyday use) for up to 1 month.

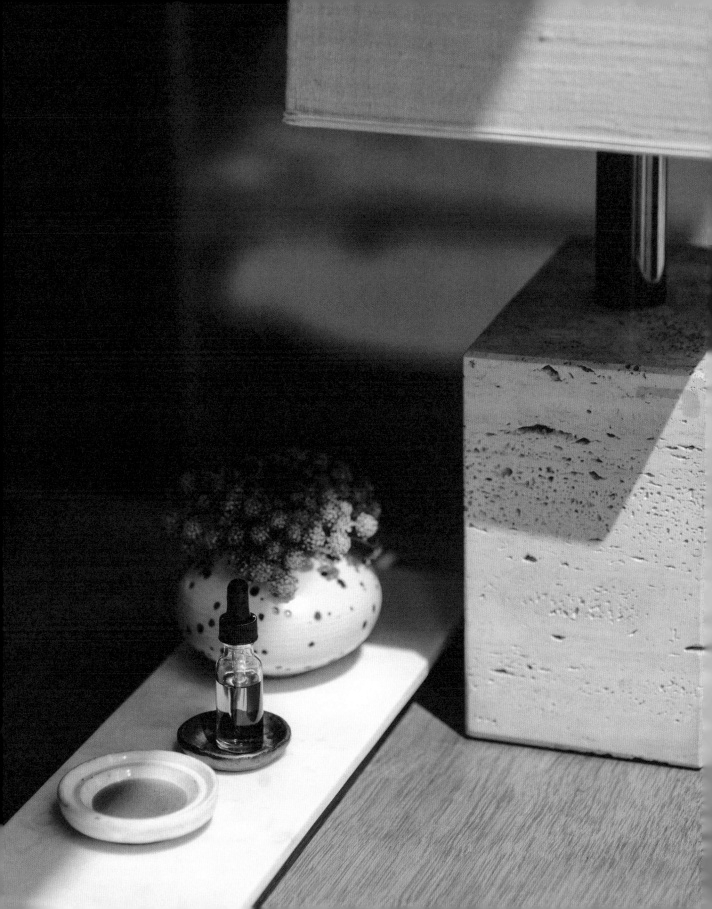

Salt Water Hair Tonic

An easy-breezy hair tonic that takes you right to the beach.

TIME: 10 minutes

MAKES: 1 ounce (30 mL) hair tonic

YOU'LL NEED: a 1-ounce (30 mL) mist bottle

COMPONENTS

1 tablespoon pink Himalayan sea salt

1 teaspoon fractionated coconut oil

10 drops lavender essential oil

8 drops peppermint essential oil

4 drops lemongrass essential oil

I have thin and fine hair, which means that every day by around 2 pm, it's a little greasy and flat. Depending on how busy my day is, my hair tends to take on the same dynamic, messy nature. This salt water hair tonic is my favourite afternoon pick-me-up for both taming fly-aways and oily roots and amplifying and adding volume. You can keep it at your desk or in your bag and reach for it whenever your hair needs a little extra *oomph*. I love keeping it in my gym bag, too—in case I end up going to a yoga or Pilates class at lunch or after work.

Sea salt tonics have become incredibly popular in the mainstream beauty industry, and they are quite expensive considering the ingredients you'll find in them. Growing up near the ocean, I always made my own sea salt spray because I never found a hair product at our local drugstore that had the same dynamic ability of true seawater to naturally improve volume and texture and decrease afternoon grease. This recipe is a more elevated version of the one I made while growing up. I've added trace amounts of fractionated (liquid) coconut oil, which help with taming fly-aways and add a slight tropical aroma. I hope this sea salt spray mentally takes you right to the beach. No matter where you are in the world or what your day is throwing at you, at least you can have carefree, surfer-inspired hair.

METHOD

1. Pour the warm water into the mist bottle and add the sea salt. Shake until most of the salt has dissolved (it's normal for not all of the salt to dissolve fully).
2. Add the fractionated coconut oil to the warm salt water mixture.
3. Add the essential oils and shake well.

APPLICATION

1. Mist the sea salt hair tonic all over dry hair for added volume and lift. If applying to damp hair, after a workout class or shower, apply all over and then scrunch hair with your hands and allow to air-dry.

STORAGE

Keep in a cool, dry place for up to 1 month.

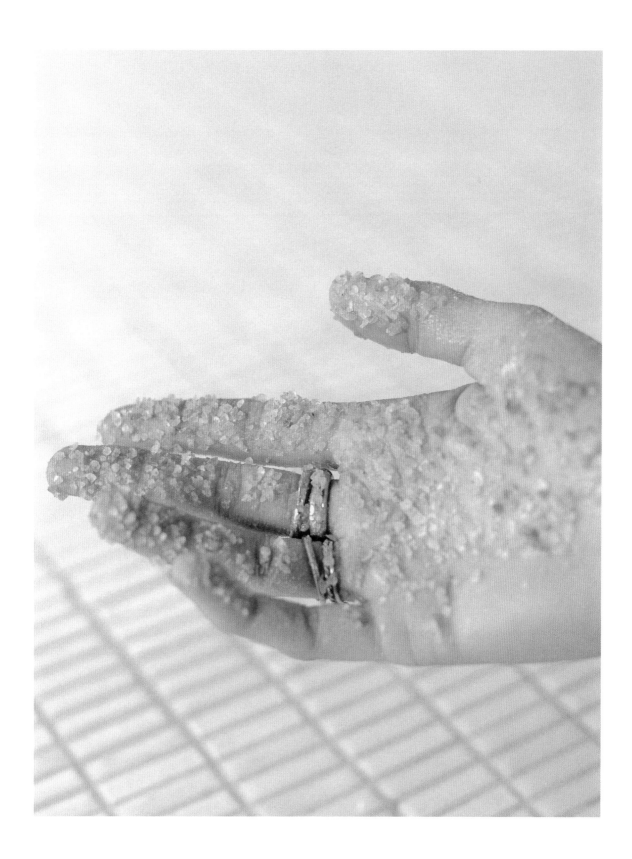

NATURAL HAIR PERFUMES

There's nothing better than a flip of the hair that smells goddess-like, healthy and full. Natural hair perfumes are a hidden secret weapon for moments of intimacy, such as a date or special event, when people may be leaning in a little closer than usual to speak to you.

Hair can sometimes hold scent better than a sweater or clothing, and the layers of scent you add to your body throughout the day can complement each other. They can even result in a dynamic and personalized aroma. The aroma of your morning face oils and the essential oils in your shower scrub may make up the first layer. The next layer comes from a quick dab of your favourite natural perfume or a roll-on product on your wrists. Finally, the last layer that adds dimension to your personal aroma is your hair. I like using hair perfume as a quick, easy way to refresh. When customizing yours, choose aromas that help you reset and feel your best in the middle of the day. I've designed these recipes with three base options you can choose from depending on your hair type.

BASE OPTIONS

WITCH HAZEL (OILY OR FINE HAIR)
Witch hazel (non-alcoholic) is a great option for fine and oily hair because it helps diffuse the properties and aroma of the essential oils throughout the hair without weighing it down. Using witch hazel as the base will result in a more lightweight product that shouldn't be used on more naturally dry hair.

JOJOBA OIL (CURLY OR DRY HAIR)
The complexity and consistency of jojoba oil naturally mimics the oil produced on the scalp, which makes it a great base to use for controlling fly-aways without making the hair look too weighed down.

NATURAL ALOE VERA GEL (NORMAL OR SUN-EXPOSED HAIR)
For a more dynamic, loose hold on the hair perfume, opt for aloe vera gel as your base. It's especially nice for hair that's exposed to warmer climates and is a nice way to add moisture without directly using oil.

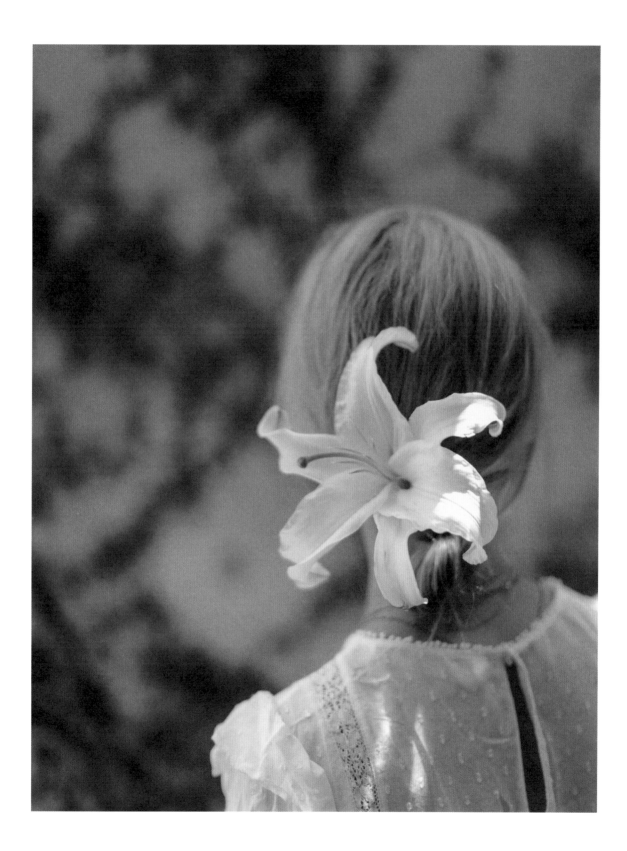

Goddess Hair Perfume

For when you want to smell amazing . . . for yourself.

TIME: 5 minutes

MAKES: 1 ounce (30 mL) hair perfume

YOU'LL NEED: a 1-ounce (30 mL) mist bottle

COMPONENTS

2 teaspoons base (see page 92)

2 tablespoons filtered water or rose water

20 drops geranium essential oil

20 drops rosemary essential oil

10 drops ylang ylang essential oil

There is something about the scent of hair that can change the way you feel about yourself. A mist of hair perfume before I go out the door makes everything feel complete. It's also a great way to feel fresh on the go while travelling—this blend of floral essential oils is my go-to hair aroma, regardless of where I am in the world. Floral aromas are energetically very powerful because of the volume of flower petals that go into making just a small amount of the oil. This energy is concentrated in the essential oil, and I'm reminded of the women centuries before me who used flower essences and essential oils in their beauty rituals.

METHOD

1. Choose the base for your hair type and add to the mist bottle.
2. Add the filtered water or rose water. Both will work, but I like using rose water because it smells lovely and feels a little more luxurious.
3. Add all the essential oils and shake well.

APPLICATION

1. Shake the mist bottle before each use.
2. Mist all over hair.
3. Breathe deeply.

STORAGE

Keep in a cool, dry place for up to 3 months.

Masculine and Spicy Hair Perfume

For when you're expecting those close-quarters moments.

TIME: 5 minutes

MAKES: 1 ounce (30 mL) hair perfume

YOU'LL NEED: a 1-ounce (30 mL) mist bottle

COMPONENTS

2 teaspoons base (see page 92)

2 tablespoons filtered water or rose water

20 drops cedarwood essential oil

20 drops rosemary essential oil

10 drops spruce essential oil

STORAGE

Keep in a cool, dry place for up to 3 months.

In the winter, adding a more dynamic and earthier aroma to the hair is a nice way to feel grounded and centred—not to mention that it adds a simple allure as you move your hair, walk past someone or get closer in those more intimate moments. This grounding hair perfume can be used by both men and women. Not only does it smell great, but the essential oils included in it are beneficial to the hair follicles and can help promote healthy hair growth. This hair perfume is really a win-win.

METHOD

1. Choose the base for your hair type and add to the mist bottle.
2. Add the filtered water or rose water. Both will work, but I like using rose water because it smells lovely and feels a little more luxurious.
3. Add all the essential oils and shake well.

APPLICATION

1. Shake the mist bottle before each use.
2. Mist all over hair.
3. Breathe deeply.

Beach Bliss Hair Perfume

For a mini beach escape that's always nearby.

TIME: 5 minutes

MAKES: 1 ounce (30 mL) hair perfume

YOU'LL NEED: a 1-ounce (30 mL) mist bottle

COMPONENTS

2 teaspoons base (see page 92)

2 tablespoons filtered water or rose water

20 drops peppermint essential oil

20 drops grapefruit essential oil

10 drops lemongrass essential oil

STORAGE

Keep in a cool, dry place for up to 3 months

Not only is the water my happy place, but I love what it does to my skin and hair. It provides naturally exfoliated skin and beach wave hair that can really only be accomplished while doing things you love in the ocean. The fresh peppermint and citrus work beautifully with the saltiness of the water to create good summer vibes.

METHOD

1. Choose the base for your hair type and add to the mist bottle.
2. Add the filtered water or rose water. Both will work, but I like using rose water because it smells lovely and feels a little more luxurious.
3. Add all the essential oils and shake well.

APPLICATION

1. Shake the mist bottle before each use.
2. Mist all over hair.
3. Breathe deeply.

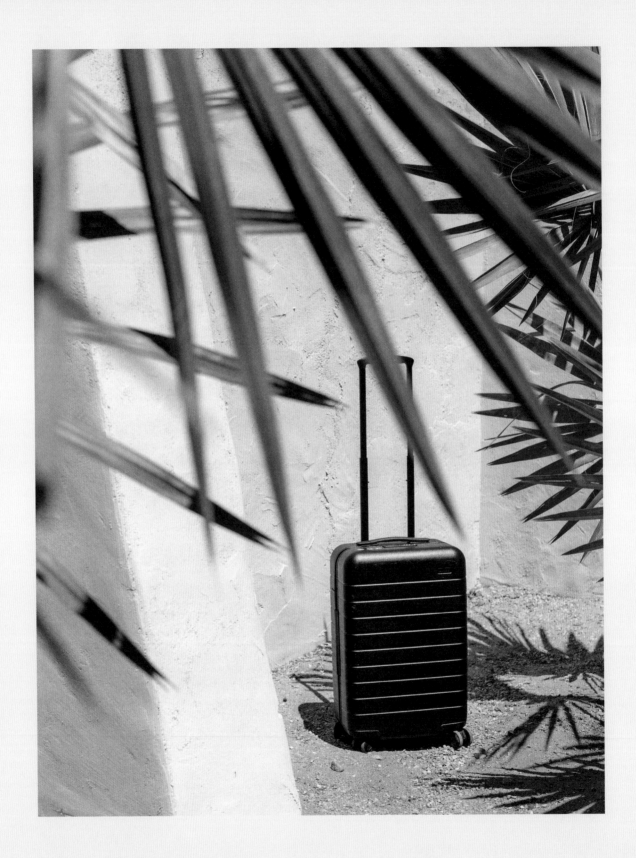

BEAUTY TRAVEL ESSENTIALS

Travelling is actually one of the times I use essential oils the most because they help me feel like there's a little piece of home with me. Wherever I am in the world, it's comforting to know I can continue my daily rituals on the road. Travelling is also a great example of how scent association works. For instance, I always rub one drop of lavender essential oil under my nose when I'm on a plane. The antibacterial properties are great for warding off germs, and the scent is soothing and calming. Now, whenever I add that drop right below my nose, my brain knows it's time to relax, and I can usually drift off to sleep. Sometimes I'll even add a drop to my sleep mask, especially if I'm travelling on a red-eye flight or have to adjust to a time change as soon as I land.

Creating your own DIY travel products is great for carry-on luggage as well, because you can control the quantities of your liquids. Whether I'm travelling for business or for fun, I always have my little homemade apothecary with me. The travel tips and recipes I share in this section are meant to help you maintain your beauty rituals while you're on the go.

Lip and Brow Balm

A moisturizing balm that covers all your bases.

TIME: 5 minutes

MAKES: 0.85 ounce (25 mL) balm

YOU'LL NEED: a double boiler and a 1-ounce (30 mL) tin or glass container

COMPONENTS

2 teaspoons organic solid virgin coconut oil

2 teaspoons organic cocoa butter

1 teaspoon organic beeswax

8 drops essential oil of your choice (I love using lavender, grapefruit or peppermint)

A multi-purpose balm is a travel essential for me. I love having something that can be used in multiple ways, and the fact that this balm can be used for hands, lips and brows makes it super easy to pack. Plus, it's not a liquid, so it's one less thing for airport security to be concerned about.

METHOD

1. In a double boiler over low heat, combine the coconut oil, cocoa butter and beeswax and stir until melted.
2. Remove from heat and continue stirring. When the mixture begins to cool, it will begin to thicken and the colour will turn milky; at this time, add the essential oils and continue stirring.
3. Pour the mixture into the container and let cool without a lid (covering it results in condensation, which prevents the balm from drying correctly). Allow the balm to cool for 6 to 8 hours (or overnight), then cover.

APPLICATION

1. Using your fingers, apply the natural balm to your lips and brows as desired throughout the day.

STORAGE

Keep in a cool, dry place (or your purse) for up to 3 months.

Cuticle Oil

A nourishing cuticle oil for 35,000 feet.

TIME: 2 minutes
MAKES: 0.5 ounce (15 mL)
cuticle oil
YOU'LL NEED: a 0.5-ounce
(15 mL) dropper bottle

COMPONENTS

1 teaspoon jojoba oil

2 teaspoons rosehip oil

3 drops lemon essential oil

1 drop frankincense essential oil

This recipe is a great pick-me-up for when travel dries out your hands and cuticles (airplanes are notorious for drying out the skin). Using a cuticle oil while I travel also helps me maintain my manicure (which is always a good thing) and tends to decrease the chipping that occurs. All you have to do is mix the ingredients in a dark glass dropper bottle.

METHOD

1. Mix all the oils in the dropper bottle.

APPLICATION

1. Apply 1 to 2 drops on dry cuticles and use your fingers to massage it into the nail beds.

STORAGE

Keep in a cool, dry place (like your purse or carry-on luggage) for up to 1 month.

Foot Soak

A little reprieve for feet that have traipsed around the city all day.

TIME: 15 minutes
MAKES: 1 foot soak
YOU'LL NEED: a bathtub

COMPONENTS

10 drops eucalyptus essential oil

10 drops sweet orange
essential oil

A foot soak is something super simple you can do when you get to your hotel after a long day of travel. All you have to do is fill your hotel bathtub with 3 inches of water, then add 10 drops of eucalyptus essential oil and 10 drops of sweet orange essential oil. While your feet soak, do some simple seated stretches to help create body awareness and quiet the mind.

METHOD AND APPLICATION

1. Fill the bathtub with 3 inches of warm water, then add the essential oils.
2. While your feet soak, do some simple seated stretches: bring your arms above your head, shift to the side and stretch your hamstrings by gently leaning forward with a straight back. Soak and stretch for 10 to 15 minutes.

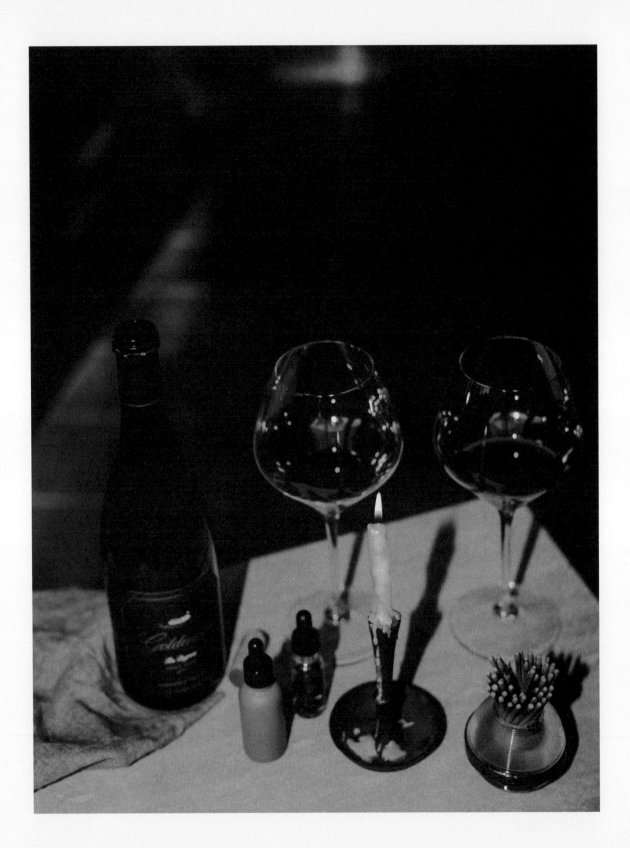

EVENING BEAUTY RITUALS

Preparing for bed is one of my favourite parts of the day. The process of cleansing and moisturizing my face and body is one of the few practices that's consistent, regardless of where I am or how hectic my day has been. An evening beauty ritual is perhaps the most sacred and calming of all—it's a chance to take a little more time for yourself, even if that's just another extra-long, luxurious minute to help you unwind.

Beyond literally removing dirt and makeup, a ritualistic evening routine can help you wash away the stress and all-consuming thoughts that have accumulated during your busy day. If you're anything like me, you might be a little more sensitive to people's energies and feel more than others might during your day—which makes the evening beauty routine even more crucial. I personally find it to be a cathartic experience. It's a chance to prepare for a fresh start tomorrow, knowing that all you have ahead of you is a new day with new possibilities. Here, I share a few of my favourite evening beauty rituals with essential oils. I hope they'll provide you with the same grounding energy they've given me, while also sending you to bed feeling a little lighter.

Gentle Hydrating Eye Makeup Remover Balm

A simple anytime, anywhere natural makeup remover.

TIME: 6 minutes

MAKES: 2 ounces (60 mL) eye makeup remover

YOU'LL NEED: a saucepan, a 2-ounce (60 mL) tin or glass container and an organic cotton face pad

COMPONENTS

2 tablespoons organic solid virgin coconut oil

2 tablespoons sweet almond oil

6 drops frankincense essential oil

Usually the first step in an evening beauty routine is removing your makeup. Although there are plenty of conventional makeup removers out there, I prefer making my own so I know all the ingredients are natural and gentle on my skin. I also love that this recipe is a "balm" rather than a water-based makeup remover. It means you can sneak in a little face massage while you're at it. The balm feels super nourishing to the skin (a well-deserved luxury after a long day), but it doesn't clog the pores. Plus, with this recipe, when I run out of the balm I have all the ingredients lying around my house, so it's easy to whip up another batch.

The properties of coconut oil make it incredibly useful for naturally breaking down makeup (including the most stubborn mascaras) and wiping your face clean. Beyond smelling amazing and being handy in the kitchen, coconut oil has naturally occurring antibacterial properties, which make it even more effective at removing dirt, makeup and bacteria that may clog pores and cause blemishes. This product is super easy to make and use and will remove most eye makeups.

METHOD

1. In a small saucepan, heat the coconut oil over low heat until fully melted. Add in the sweet almond oil and stir to combine.
2. When the mixture is warm and fully combined, pour it into a tin or glass container.
3. As the mixture begins to cool (you will see it start to turn a slightly milky colour), add the frankincense essential oil to the container.
4. Leave the container uncovered until all moisture is evaporated and the balm is fully cooled.

APPLICATION

1. Using your finger or a small spoon, scoop about 1 teaspoon of the balm into your hand and warm it between your fingers.
2. Apply the balm over the eyelid and around the eyes. Massage it into the face, starting at the brow, then moving to the upper cheekbone and in toward the nose.
3. To remove any remaining eye makeup, warm the oil with your fingers and apply it to a cotton face pad. Apply the face pad to the eyes to remove mascara, then use warm water to help remove any leftover balm.

STORAGE

Keep in a tin or glass container, covered, in your bathroom away from direct sunlight for up to 2 weeks.

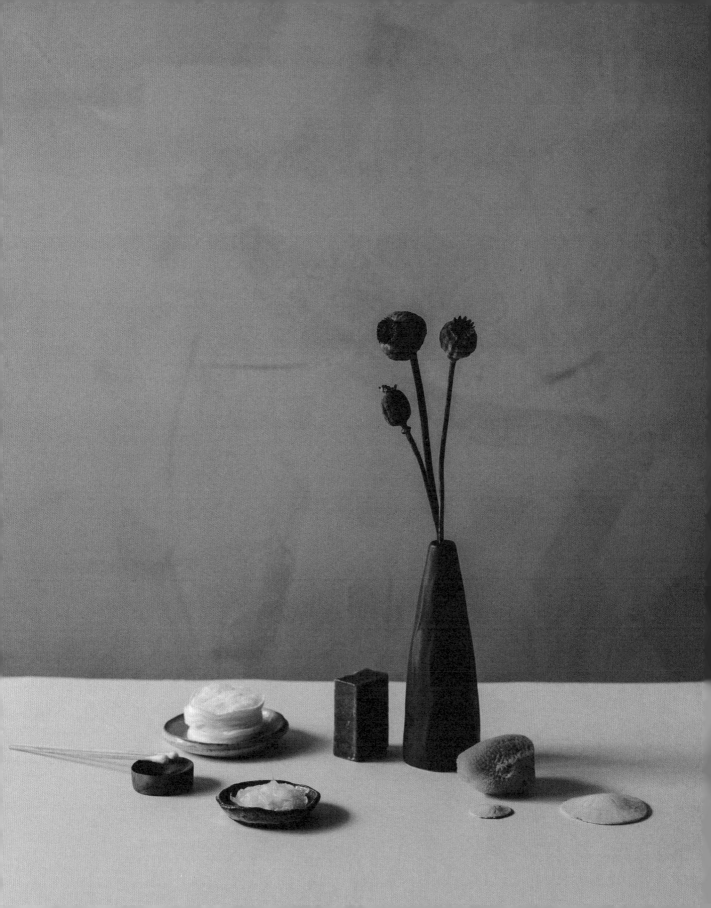

EVENING FACE OIL CLEANSERS

Cleansers are my favourite product to make myself. A good cleanser should be gentle on the skin and remove all dirt and makeup, while also leaving the natural moisture of the skin intact. Soap-based cleansers can strip the skin of its natural oils and sebum (oil secreted by the body's sebaceous glands), causing the skin to overproduce oil, which can lead to blemishes, oily spots and even dry patches with excessive use. Many of us have gotten used to that "squeaky clean" feeling of a soap-based cleanser, but the astringent properties can be counterproductive in the long run, and I much prefer using an oil cleanser. The following cleansers are easy to make and cost effective. I don't spend my beauty budget on fancy cleansers because a cleanser is really used to prep the skin for the more effective products that follow it. I prefer to keep things simple when it comes to cleansing, then invest in creating more dynamic serums and face oils that I apply before bed—giving them all evening (or as many hours of sleep as I can get) to work their magic.

You'll notice that all but one of these recipes include coconut oil—that's because it has incredible moisturizing properties that leave the skin smooth and protected. I also love using coconut oil because its anti-inflammatory and soothing properties can help decrease redness and inflammation and its anti-bacterial benefits help clean out pores, as well as prevent blemishes.

Rosehip oil is also included in most of these recipes because it is very high in antioxidants, which is a great addition to a cleanser—especially if you want to get more benefits from your cleanser before applying your face oil and serums.

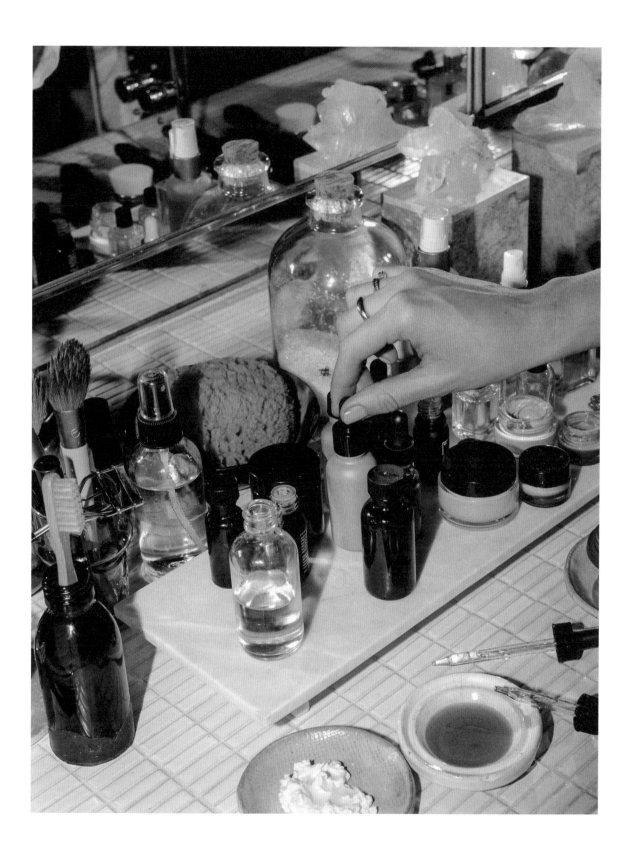

Calming Lavender and Coconut Face Oil Cleanser (Sensitive Skin)

A soothing cleanser that can help you chill out before bed.

TIME: 5 minutes

MAKES: 1 ounce (30 mL) cleanser

YOU'LL NEED: a small bowl and a face cloth

COMPONENTS

1 tablespoon organic solid virgin coconut oil

1 tablespoon jojoba oil

3 drops lavender essential oil

This gentle oil cleanser is great for those with sensitive skin. It can be used day and night, but I especially love it for evenings because the herbal lavender paired with the lightly sweet coconut oil gives off an incredibly soothing aroma that prepares your mind for bed. Plus, the lavender and coconut oil both have gentle antimicrobial properties, so I know the dirt is effectively being removed from my skin. I also use this cleanser if my face is feeling oversensitive or if I have redness from extensive travel or stress. It's a nice, simple go-to oil cleanser for anytime you need to be gentle to your face.

METHOD

1. In a small bowl, mix together all components until the coconut oil is incorporated. You may need to melt the coconut oil slightly before mixing by placing the closed coconut oil jar under hot water for 1 or 2 minutes.

APPLICATION

1. Apply 1 teaspoon of face oil cleanser to the hands and then using your fingers apply it to the face, being careful to avoid the eyes.
2. Massage in an outward direction using small circular movements. While doing so, take long, deep breaths as the coconut oil melts into the face.
3. Continue making circular outward movements on the face, starting at the nose, moving to the forehead and finishing with the chin and neck (often forgotten).
4. To remove the cleanser, add very warm water to a clean face cloth (I prefer organic cotton or bamboo) and wipe the face clean. If necessary, rewarm the face cloth with water to create a fresh cloth and continue to wipe away any excess cleanser.

STORAGE

Keep in a cool, dry place away from direct sunlight for up to 2 weeks.

Ultra-Moisturizing Avocado Face Oil Cleanser (Dry Skin)

A nourishing cleanser that locks in moisture.

TIME: 5 minutes

MAKES: 1.35 ounces (40 mL) cleanser

YOU'LL NEED: a small bowl and a face cloth

COMPONENTS

2 teaspoons organic solid virgin coconut oil

2 teaspoons avocado oil

2 teaspoons rosehip oil

3 drops frankincense essential oil

Adding an oil cleanser to your routine can be a game changer for those with dry skin. Not only will it leave your skin feeling more hydrated and nourished, it's also gentler and far less irritating than traditional cleansers, which is incredibly important for those with dry skin. I love using this deeply nourishing oil cleanser when my skin is dry in the winter because it leaves my face feeling clean yet sealed in with moisture.

METHOD

1. In a small bowl, mix together all components until the coconut oil is incorporated. You may need to melt the coconut oil slightly before mixing by placing the closed coconut oil jar under hot water for 1 or 2 minutes.

APPLICATION

1. Apply 1 teaspoon of face oil cleanser to the hands and then using your fingers apply it to the face, being careful to avoid the eyes.
2. Massage in an outward direction using small circular movements. While doing so, take long, deep breaths as the coconut oil melts into the face.
3. Continue making circular outward movements on the face, starting at the nose, moving to the forehead and finishing with the chin and neck (often forgotten).
4. To remove the cleanser, add very warm water to a clean face cloth (I prefer organic cotton or bamboo) and wipe the face clean. If necessary, rewarm the face cloth with water to create a fresh cloth and continue to wipe away any excess cleanser.

STORAGE

Keep in a cool, dry place away from direct sunlight for up to 2 weeks.

Lightweight Grapeseed and Rosehip Face Oil Cleanser (Oily Skin)

A hydrating yet fresh cleanser that fights oil with oil.

TIME: 5 minutes

MAKES: 1 ounce (30 mL) cleanser

YOU'LL NEED: a small bowl and a face cloth

COMPONENTS

2 teaspoons organic solid virgin coconut oil

2 teaspoons rosehip oil

2 teaspoons grapeseed oil

2 drops lavender essential oil

1 drop tea tree essential oil

Your skin is most likely overproducing oil because it lacks it, so by introducing an oil cleanser, you're really giving the skin what it needs and wants. I like to use this cleanser when I've been travelling all day and my skin is feeling oily from pollution, stale airplane air or overall stress. In this recipe, I've added tea tree and lavender essential oils to the coconut oil because they naturally boost the antibacterial and antimicrobial properties of the coconut oil and help prevent blemishes. I love using a cleanser that's as active as this because it leaves the skin tingling and fresh.

METHOD

1. In a small bowl, mix together all components until the coconut oil is incorporated. You may need to melt the coconut oil slightly before mixing by placing the closed coconut oil jar under hot water for 1 or 2 minutes.

APPLICATION

1. Apply 1 teaspoon of face oil cleanser to the hands and then using your fingers apply it to the face, being careful to avoid the eyes.
2. Massage in an outward direction using small circular movements. While doing so, take long, deep breaths as the coconut oil melts into the face.
3. Continue making circular outward movements on the face, starting at the nose, moving to the forehead and finishing with the chin and neck (often forgotten).
4. To remove the cleanser, add very warm water to a clean face cloth (I prefer organic cotton or bamboo) and wipe the face clean. If necessary, rewarm the face cloth with water to create a fresh cloth and continue to wipe away any excess cleanser.

STORAGE

Keep in a cool, dry place away from direct sunlight for up to 2 weeks.

Balancing Geranium and Jojoba Face Oil Cleanser (Combination Skin)

A gentle cleanser that truly has the balancing act figured out.

TIME: 5 minutes

MAKES: 1 ounce (30 mL) cleanser

YOU'LL NEED: a small bowl and a face cloth

COMPONENTS

3 teaspoons organic solid virgin coconut oil

3 teaspoons jojoba oil

2 drops geranium essential oil

2 drops sweet orange essential oil

The goal with combination skin is always to find balance, which can be tricky. In this recipe, I've included what I consider to be a pretty dynamic duo: geranium and sweet orange essential oils. Both are gentle and balancing for the skin, which make them great components for an everyday cleanser. Geranium is one of my favourite scents—it's soft and feminine—while the sweet orange is bright and invigorating. Using this day or night will refresh and reset your face and mood.

METHOD

1. In a small bowl, mix together all components until the coconut oil is incorporated. You may need to melt the coconut oil slightly before mixing by placing the closed coconut oil jar under hot water for 1 or 2 minutes.

APPLICATION

1. Apply 1 teaspoon of face oil cleanser to the hands and then using your fingers apply it to the face, being careful to avoid the eyes.
2. Massage in an outward direction using small circular movements. While doing so, take long, deep breaths as the coconut oil melts into the face.
3. Continue making circular outward movements on the face, starting at the nose, moving to the forehead and finishing with the chin and neck (often forgotten).
4. To remove the cleanser, add very warm water to a clean face cloth (I prefer organic cotton or bamboo) and wipe the face clean. If necessary, rewarm the face cloth with water to create a fresh cloth and continue to wipe away any excess cleanser.

STORAGE

Keep in a cool, dry place away from direct sunlight for up to 2 weeks.

Nourishing Frankincense and Ylang Ylang Face Oil Cleanser (Mature Skin)

A super-hydrating cleanser for when your skin needs a little boost.

TIME: 5 minutes

MAKES: 1 ounce (30 mL) cleanser

YOU'LL NEED: a 1-ounce (30 mL) dropper bottle and a face cloth

COMPONENTS

3 teaspoons avocado oil

3 teaspoons rosehip oil

2 drops frankincense essential oil

1 drop ylang ylang essential oil

For mature skin, I love designing nourishing and ultra-hydrating cleansers that provide a feeling of satin on the skin and have a consistency that's easy to massage into the face. This rich cleansing oil is a favourite for those with mature skin or for anyone who has skin that's craving something really nourishing.

METHOD

1. Mix together all components in a dropper bottle.

APPLICATION

1. Apply 1 teaspoon of face oil cleanser to the hands and then using your fingers apply it to the face, being careful to avoid the eyes.
2. Massage in an outward direction using small circular movements. While doing so, take long, deep breaths.
3. Continue making circular outward movements on the face, starting at the nose, moving to the forehead and finishing with the chin and neck (often forgotten).
4. To remove the cleanser, add very warm water to a clean face cloth (I prefer organic cotton or bamboo) and wipe the face clean. If necessary, rewarm the face cloth with water to create a fresh cloth and continue to wipe away any excess cleanser.

STORAGE

Keep in a cool, dry place away from direct sunlight for up to 2 weeks.

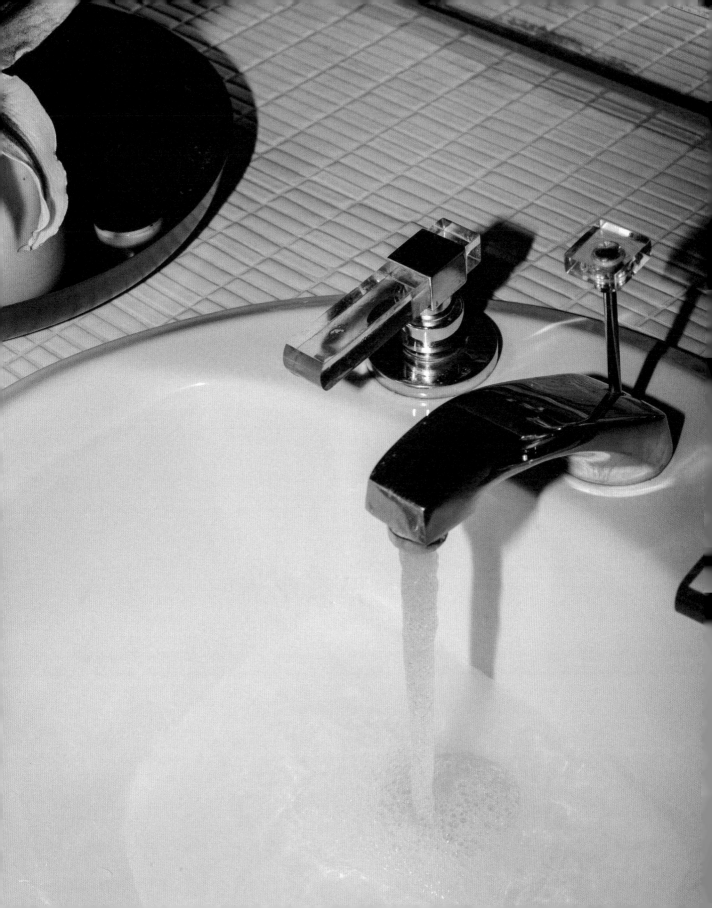

EVENING FACE STEAMS

Face steams are the simplest way to bring the spa into your home, and they take much less prep and cleanup time than you probably think. The benefit of doing a face steam after cleansing is that the hot water helps open the pores and removes a layer of dirt, bacteria and buildup from the face. The hot water also heats the essential oils and causes them to evaporate. These face steams are designed to trap those evaporated essential oils and guide them into the open pores, so that you experience their benefits in the most direct way possible.

The steam and intensity of the hot water also help open the lungs and respiratory passages—one of the reasons I love doing this practice on a Friday evening after a very long week. My nose, airways and respiratory system feel cleansed and rejuvenated after a steam. There's something about "clearing out all the stuff," both literally and figuratively, at the end of a week that I really need sometimes.

Because of the added respiratory benefits, I try to do two to three face steams per week during cold and flu season. I usually use a mix of tea tree and lavender essential oils because it helps cleanse the pores while also providing added antimicrobial and antibacterial benefits throughout the respiratory tract.

Although this may not be an "every evening" type of experience for you in your jam-packed days, I try to fit in a face steam on Friday evenings (even if I'm super exhausted), as well as on Sunday evenings. They help me ease into the weekend or the start of a new workweek feeling cleansed.

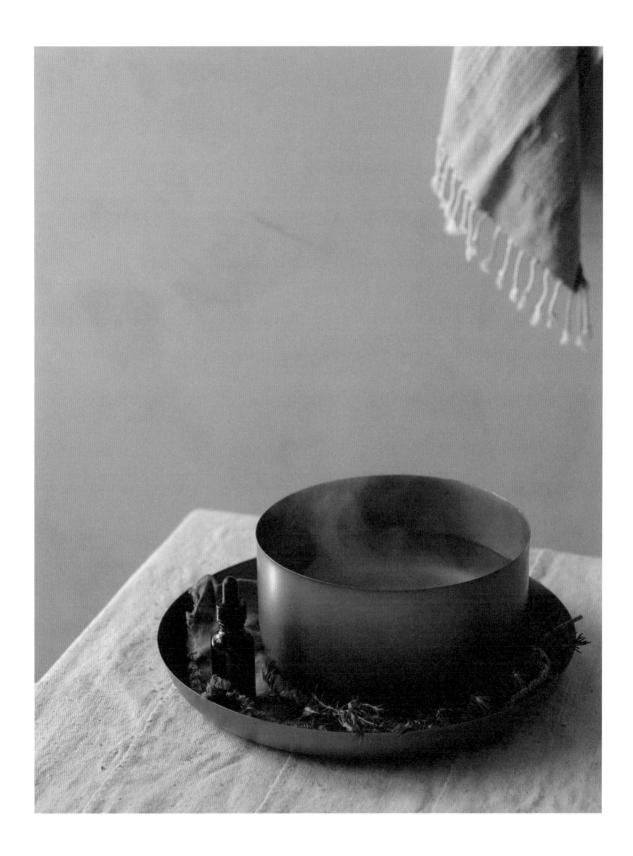

Hydrating Face Steam

A grounding face steam that's perfect at the end of a long day.

TIME: 15 minutes

MAKES: 1 face steam

YOU'LL NEED: a large bowl (to steam the whole face) and a large towel (to cover your head over the bowl)

COMPONENTS

Boiling filtered water

3 drops geranium essential oil

3 drops frankincense essential oil

This is my go-to face steam for when I want something calming on the skin and need some extra hydration before bed. Geranium essential oil has a floral aroma with a slightly minty-fresh undertone, making it perfectly goddess-like and refreshing for a facial steam. Geranium essential oils and flowers have been used for centuries to balance and tone the skin and can be beneficial for toning skin changes that are due to hormonal imbalances. Frankincense is lovely to use for an evening face steam because the resinous aroma is incredibly grounding and calming.

METHOD

1. Fill a large bowl with boiling water set on a countertop or kitchen table. You can place a bath towel under the bowl to protect the surface and keep it from sliding around.
2. Add the essential oils to the hot water.
3. Sit or stand with your face over the bowl and drape the towel over your head. Make sure to keep all the steam under the towel so it doesn't escape.
4. Close your eyes and steam your face for 1 to 4 minutes.
5. Breathe deeply and know you took a moment to do something good for yourself (and your skin).

Cleansing Face Steam

A refreshing face steam that clears your skin and opens your airways.

TIME: 15 minutes

MAKES: 1 face steam

YOU'LL NEED: a large bowl (to steam the whole face) and a large towel (to cover your head over the bowl)

COMPONENTS

Boiling filtered water

2 drops lavender essential oil

1 drop lemongrass essential oil

1 drop tea tree essential oil

This recipe is a great option for when your skin feels backed up and bloated and needs a deep clean. I love using this face steam during the winter months, when I'm wearing a little more makeup and using richer face products in an attempt to seal in moisture. This ultra-refreshing, cleansing face steam is also my go-to during cold and flu season, when I want my respiratory tract to experience the benefits of the antibacterial and antimicrobial properties of lavender and tea tree essential oils. With this face steam, it's extra important to keep your eyes closed because the volatile oils and qualities of tea tree can be intense and irritating to the eyes when heated. I hope you enjoy the refreshing benefits of this face steam as much as I do.

METHOD

1. Fill a large bowl with boiling water set on a countertop or kitchen table. You can place a bath towel under the bowl to protect the surface and keep it from sliding around.
2. Add the essential oils to the hot water.
3. Sit or stand with your face over the bowl and drape the towel over your head. Make sure to keep all the steam under the towel so it doesn't escape.
4. Close your eyes and steam your face for 1 to 4 minutes.
5. Breathe deeply and know you took a moment to do something good for yourself (and your skin).

FACE MASKS

There's perhaps nothing more quintessentially luxurious than a face mask in the evening. In fact, it's not even considered weird anymore to cancel your Friday night plans in favour of staying home and "masking." For me, the ritual of applying it, the inability to leave your home while you're wearing it and the feeling that you've added another layer of productivity to your already dynamic life are what make me a face mask fan. And, in all honesty, approximately 70 percent of this book was written while wearing a face mask, so these words are proof that masking can be productive.

Throughout my life, a face mask has been the reward and nudge of self-care I need to finish a long day. It's the ritual that brings me right over the finish line. I've often bribed myself to finish late-night emails with the knowledge that I'll do it when I have a mask on, with a cup of my favourite green tea. Our company is all about "elevating the simple moments," and this is something I've definitely done with a face mask on many occasions.

I truly hope you enjoy these face mask recipes with the same amount of presence and feeling of self-care that I do. They're one of my favourite ways to unwind and finish the day, and they all take less than 5 minutes to make. Masking is a beauty ritual that's doable any day of the week, whenever you need an extra-luxurious yet incredibly simple moment of "you time."

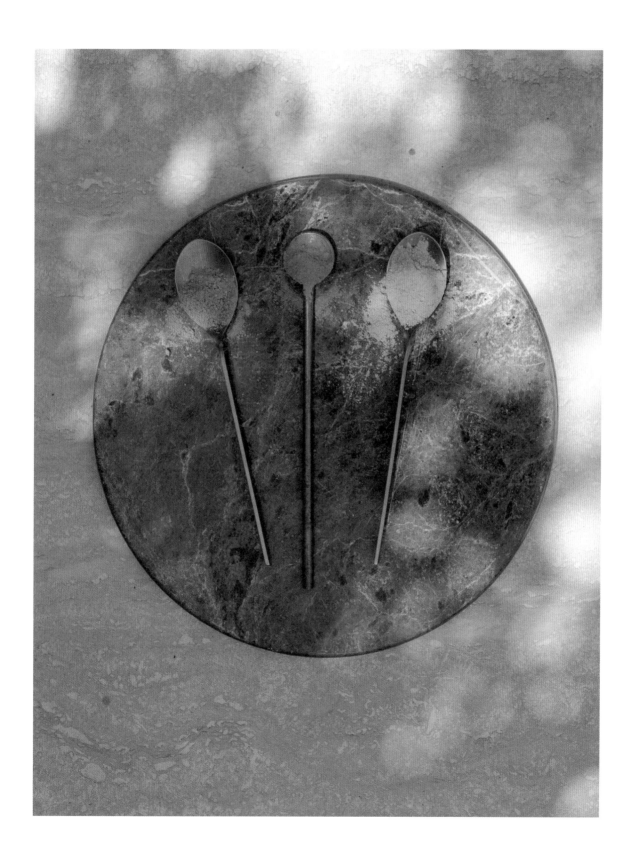

Honey and Lavender Oil-Balancing Face Mask

A face mask that smells as lovely as it sounds.

TIME: 2 minutes to make, best left on for 20 minutes

MAKES: 1 face mask

YOU'LL NEED: a small bowl, a metal spoon and 2 face cloths

COMPONENTS

1 tablespoon organic liquid honey

1 tablespoon sweet almond oil

2 drops bergamot essential oil

2 drops lavender essential oil

1 tablespoon facial clay (I use French green or pink clay)

Filtered water, as needed

This face mask is a favourite when my skin is feeling oily but still craving extra nourishment. The honey creates a beautiful texture and adds another dimension of antibacterial properties, while the sweet almond oil is soothing and nourishing. The facial clay helps pull out dirt and naturally controls oil, which leaves you with skin that feels balanced but not overly dry. The bergamot essential oil in this blend is a fresh yet calming citrus, which is great for evenings. I also included lavender essential oil because of its gentle astringent and anti-bacterial properties, which help the clay to bring its benefits directly into the pores. Each of the essential oils and ingredients was chosen with the idea of applying this mask in the evening before bed—they're comforting and soothing yet highly effective.

METHOD

1. In a small bowl, combine the honey and sweet almond oil. Stir with a metal spoon until smooth (wooden spoons stick to the honey too much).
2. Add the essential oils and continue stirring.
3. Slowly add the facial clay in small amounts, stirring to maintain a smooth consistency.
4. If needed, add the water 1 teaspoon at a time to reach a smooth yet firm consistency that you'll be able to spread on the skin without it being too thin or too liquid.

APPLICATION

1. Using a spoon or your fingers, apply the mask on the face 1 teaspoon at a time, starting at the centre and working out toward the hairline. Apply the mask under the chin and jawline, as these are areas where breakouts can also occur.
2. Allow the mask to stay on until dry, about 20 minutes (drink tea, stretch, read a book you love or finish replying to the emails in your inbox).
3. To remove, soften the mask by lightly pressing a damp, warm face cloth against the face. Then use the face cloth to remove the mask, rinsing the cloth as necessary.
4. Splash the face with water and dry with a clean face cloth to remove any leftover clay.

STORAGE

Keep any extra face mask in an airtight container in the fridge for up to 1 week. It's important to keep the face mask away from air so it doesn't dry out.

Soothing Creamy Floral Face Mask

A face mask that pairs perfectly with a glass of wine.

TIME: 2 minutes to make, best left on for 20 minutes

MAKES: 1 face mask

YOU'LL NEED: a small bowl, a metal spoon and 2 face cloths

COMPONENTS

1 tablespoon plain full-fat yogurt (dairy or dairy-free)

1 tablespoon organic liquid honey

3 drops geranium essential oil

1 tablespoon quick oats or oat flour

Filtered water, as needed

For a complete goddess-like experience, I make this mask and enjoy a cup of tea or a glass of wine while I'm wearing it. Simple yet effective, it smells so good you'll want to eat it (but don't), and it'll keep your face looking full, healthy and calm, regardless of what the world is throwing at you. I use this mask year-round—in the winter the oats and honey are hydrating and nourishing, while in the summer the yogurt is cooling and refreshing.

Geranium has a beautiful way of balancing the skin, and the yogurt and honey are dynamic ingredients that are beneficial to the skin all year round. The floral and fresh aroma of this creamy mask makes it feel extra luxurious, and I often look forward to applying it on a Friday evening to smooth away everything the week has brought.

METHOD

1. In a small bowl, combine the yogurt and honey. Stir with a metal spoon until smooth (wooden spoons stick to the honey too much).
2. Add the geranium essential oil and continue stirring.
3. Slowly add the quick oats in small amounts, stirring to maintain a smooth consistency.
4. If needed, add the water 1 teaspoon at a time to reach a smooth yet firm consistency that you'll be able to spread on the skin without it being too thin or too liquid.

APPLICATION

1. Using a spoon or your fingers, apply the mask on the face 1 teaspoon at a time, starting at the centre and working out toward the hairline. Apply the mask under the chin and jawline, as these are areas where breakouts can also occur.
2. Allow the mask to stay on until dry, about 20 minutes (drink tea, stretch, read a book you love or finish replying to the emails in your inbox).
3. To remove, soften the mask by lightly pressing a damp, warm face cloth against the face. Then use the face cloth to remove the mask, rinsing the cloth as necessary.
4. Splash the face with water and dry with a clean face cloth to remove any leftover mask.

STORAGE

Keep any extra face mask in an airtight container in the fridge for up to 1 week. It's important to keep the face mask away from air so it doesn't dry out.

Simple Purifying Matcha Face Mask

A face mask that's worth cancelling your Friday night plans for.

TIME: 2 minutes to make, best left on for 20 minutes
MAKES: 1 face mask
YOU'LL NEED: a small bowl, a spoon and 2 face cloths

COMPONENTS

1 tablespoon organic matcha

1 drop lemongrass essential oil

Filtered water, as needed

Be warned—this mask is extra alarming because of its bright green hue. It's best enjoyed, in true Japanese spirit, when home alone with a cup of green tea before bed. I love doing this mask when my skin is slightly more oily and I'm feeling like I need a fresh start. Do you know that feeling? When you just feel a little *dull*? I drink a bunch of lemon water, sip on some green tea, have fresh fruit and a simple dinner, tidy up my space and put on this mask. It's sort of a full evening detox—face, space and all.

I include lemongrass essential oil in this recipe because it's soothing and creates a spa-like atmosphere. While matcha is known for its detoxing and energizing effects internally, it also has similar benefits topically. The caffeine can help create a healthy glow, whereas the matcha itself functions like a clay to control oil, without being drying to the skin. I hope this mask and experience offers you a refreshing start—one that only true simplification can provide.

METHOD

1. Using a spoon, mix together the matcha and lemongrass essential oil in a small bowl. Add the water, 1 teaspoon at a time, until the mask becomes a smooth paste.

APPLICATION

1. Using a spoon or your fingers, apply the mask on the face 1 teaspoon at a time, starting at the centre and working out toward the hairline. Also apply to the jawline, under the chin and on the neck for extra antioxidant treatment in areas that get a lot of sun exposure.
2. Allow the mask to stay on until dry, about 20 minutes (drink tea, stretch, read a book you love or finish replying to the emails in your inbox).
3. To remove, soften the mask by lightly pressing a damp, warm face cloth against the face. Then use the face cloth to remove the mask, rinsing the cloth as necessary.
4. Splash the face with water and dry with a clean face cloth to remove any leftover mask.

STORAGE

Keep any extra face mask in an airtight container in the fridge for up to 1 week. It's important to keep the face mask away from air so it doesn't dry out.

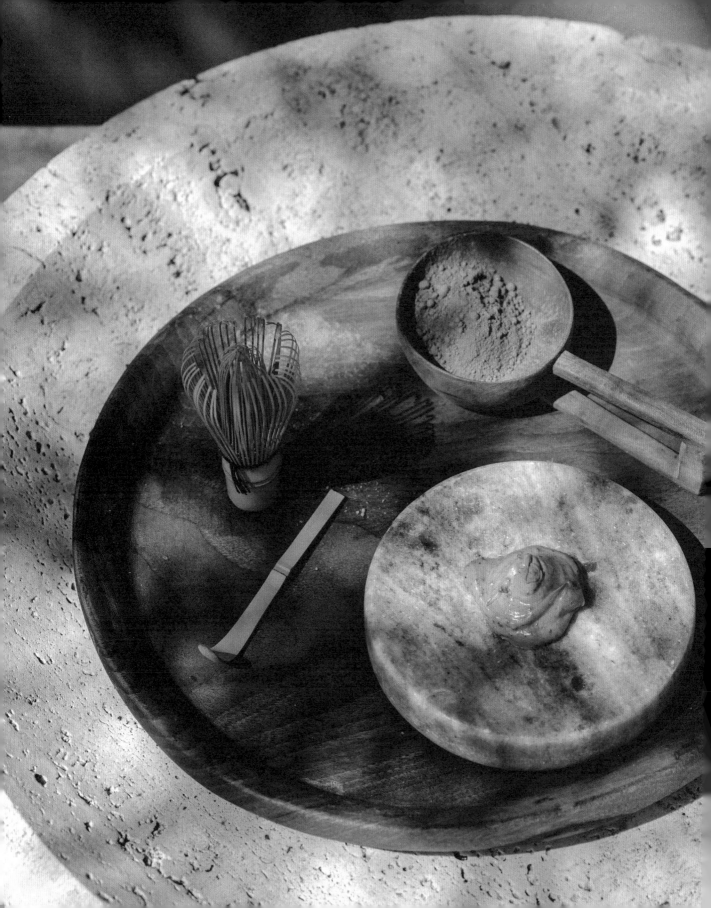

UNDER EYE SERUMS

My evening routine isn't complete without a moisture-rich serum applied to the area around my eyes. The tissue around the eye and eyelid is some of the thinnest and most sensitive on your body. This means it can often look dark and fatigued when you're experiencing lack of sleep or too much time spent in front of a computer (something I am guilty of on an almost-daily basis). What's hopeful and helpful to know about the eye area is that this thin skin is also able to absorb the benefits of natural products and essential oils very easily.

Looking at computer screens, squinting at reports, travelling, taking care of a family—all these parts of daily life are a recipe for fatigue that will, without question, show up around your eyes. There's perhaps nothing more spa-like than a well-designed and custom-blended nourishing eye serum, and after many late nights and early meetings, I want to share three of my favourite recipes. Hopefully they provide you with enough ways to get respite for your eyes at any given moment. For an extra 5 minutes of spa-like bliss, I've paired each serum with a complementary tea eye mask. These combinations should leave you feeling relaxed and nourished before bed (regardless of the amount of sleep you're about to get).

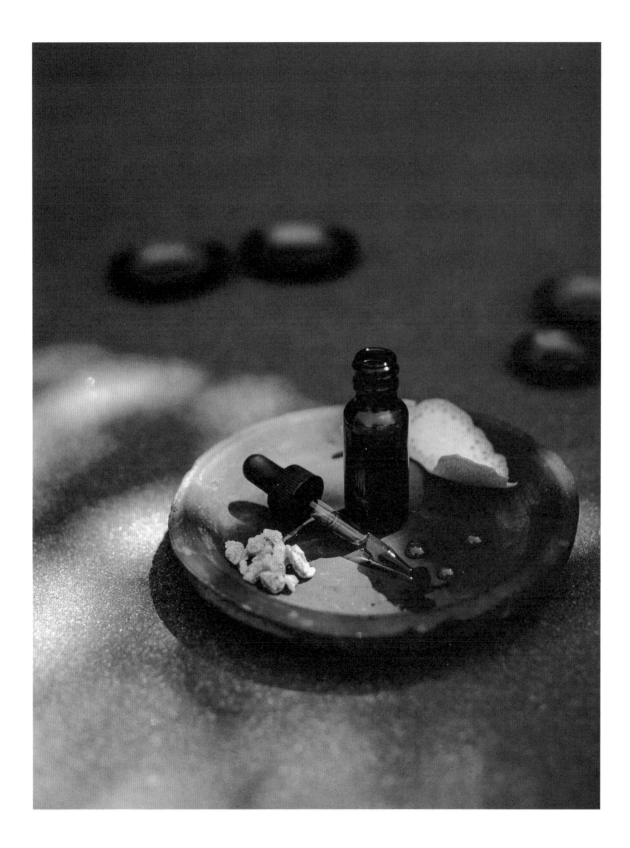

Hydrating Eye Serum with Rooibos Tea Eye Mask

An eye serum for tired, well-travelled eyes that have seen the world.

TIME: 20 minutes

MAKES: 0.67 ounce (20 mL) eye serum

YOU'LL NEED: a 1-ounce (30 mL) dropper bottle

COMPONENTS

2 teaspoons avocado oil

2 teaspoons pomegranate seed oil

2 drops frankincense essential oil

2 rooibos tea bags

Boiling filtered water

STORAGE

Keep any extra eye serum in the fridge for refreshing results or in a cool, dark place away from direct sunlight for up to 1 month.

One of my favourite eye treatments to use while travelling, this easy-to-create eye serum and tea mask combo is always in my carry-on bag. In fact, it's often the first thing I'll do when I get to a hotel. The components of this recipe have become part of my "wellness emergency kit" while travelling, and I love the relief my skin feels from the serum paired with the tea treatment. Rooibos tea is often considered an herbal alternative to chai tea because it's a warming tea without caffeine. This makes it a great choice for a hydrating eye treatment because the warmth of it paired with the serum helps prime and prep the eyes for absorbing the benefits of the oils. For the actual eye serum, I love using avocado oil with mature skin because it's one of the most hydrating base oils and sinks into the skin to promote deep hydration and plumping with its abundance of omega-3 and omega-6 fatty acids. Frankincense essential oil is the final piece in the oil mixture because it's lovely for hydration. A resin in its original form, the sap-like nature of frankincense and its traditional use in ceremonies for centuries make it one of my go-to essential oils for hydration and anything beauty ritual–related for the evening. You can make a half-batch of the eye serum for one-time use if you don't want to store any remaining product.

METHOD

1. Mix together the avocado oil, pomegranate seed oil and frankincense essential oil in a dropper bottle and gently shake to combine.
2. Pour 1 teaspoon of boiling water on each tea bag or quickly dip the tea bags in a cup of boiling water.
3. Put damp tea bags in the fridge to cool for 5 minutes.

APPLICATION

1. For best results, begin by lying down on a couch or bed (or the floor) with a pillow supporting your neck. Get comfortable with a blanket or put on some cozy clothing of your choice.
2. Close your eyes and place the 2 cooled rooibos tea bags on your eyelids.
3. For even better results, place your left hand on your chest and your right hand on your lower abdomen. Practise deep belly breathing by inhaling and pushing your lower abdomen out into your hand, then exhaling and feeling the hand fall back down and the chest rise slightly. Repeat until you can feel your energy shift and know that you've taken some deep cleansing breaths.
4. After 5 to 10 minutes of applying the tea eye mask and belly breathing, remove the tea bags.
5. Apply 1 drop of serum below each eye with your ring finger. To massage it in, lightly trace your fingers in a fluid, semicircle motion, starting at the brow and moving out toward the temple and back under the eye toward the nose. Repeat as necessary.

Toning Eye Serum with Green Tea Eye Mask

An eye serum that takes you from night to late night.

TIME: 20 minutes

MAKES: 0.67 ounce (20 mL) eye serum

YOU'LL NEED: a 1-ounce (30 mL) dropper bottle

COMPONENTS

2 teaspoons rosehip oil

2 teaspoons pomegranate seed oil

1 drop lemon essential oil

1 drop rosemary essential oil

2 organic green tea bags

Boiling filtered water

When the day has taken all the life out of your face and you need a little pick-me-up before the second shift begins, reach for this combination. This tea mask and eye serum combo is light and refreshing enough to be done before going to a dinner party or event but is effective and simple enough that it can become a part of your evening prep ritual. The lemon and rosemary essential oils give a fresh and detoxifying feeling, while the green tea eye mask gives your skin the toning and tightening feeling that only a natural astringent like green tea can. To enjoy this experience fully (especially before going out), I apply the eye mask portion of this treatment with my feet up. You can make a half-batch of the eye serum for one-time use if you don't want to store any remaining product.

METHOD

1. Mix together the rosehip oil, pomegranate seed oil, lemon essential oil and rosemary essential oil in a dropper bottle.
2. Pour 1 teaspoon of boiling water on each tea bag or quickly dip the tea bags in a cup of boiling water.
3. Put damp tea bags in the fridge to cool for 5 minutes.

APPLICATION

1. For best results, begin by lying down on a couch or bed (or the floor) with a pillow supporting your neck. Get comfortable with a blanket or put on some cozy clothing of your choice.
2. Close your eyes and place the 2 cooled green tea bags on your eyelids.
3. For even better results, place your left hand on your chest and your right hand on your lower abdomen. Practise deep belly breathing by inhaling and pushing your lower abdomen out into your hand, then exhaling and feeling the hand fall back down and the chest rise slightly. Repeat until you can feel your energy shift and know that you've taken some deep cleansing breaths.
4. After 5 to 10 minutes of applying the tea eye mask and belly breathing, remove the tea bags.
5. Apply 1 drop of serum below each eye with your ring finger. To massage it in, lightly trace your fingers in a fluid, semicircle motion, starting at the brow and moving out toward the temple and back under the eye toward the nose. Repeat as necessary.

STORAGE

Keep any extra eye serum in the fridge for refreshing results or in a cool, dark place away from direct sunlight for up to 1 month.

Calming Eye Serum with Chamomile Tea Eye Mask

An easy eye serum for when you need to make a quick recovery.

TIME: 20 minutes

MAKES: 0.67 ounce (20 mL) eye serum

YOU'LL NEED: a 1-ounce (30 mL) dropper bottle

COMPONENTS

2 teaspoons pomegranate seed oil

2 teaspoons evening primrose oil

2 drops lavender essential oil

2 organic chamomile tea bags

Boiling filtered water

I've used this eye serum and tea treatment many times after a good cry, a long night or a red-eye flight that left my eyes puffy and red. I include lavender essential oil in this recipe because of its soothing and anti-inflammatory properties. Chamomile also helps with redness and puffiness, and it's one of the most gentle botanicals you can use on your skin. Together, the lavender and chamomile help ease the eyes (and the mind). Drinking the tea itself is also a nice way to further calm any nerves. As a reminder, I recommend keeping some cooled chamomile tea bags in your fridge or freezer, so you can reach for them anytime one of "those" evenings happen. You can make a half-batch of the eye serum for one-time use if you don't want to store any remaining product.

METHOD

1. Mix together the pomegranate seed oil, sea buckthorn oil and lavender essential oil in a dropper bottle.
2. Pour 1 teaspoon of boiling water on each tea bag or quickly dip the tea bags in a cup of boiling water.
3. Put damp tea bags in the fridge to cool for 5 minutes.

APPLICATION

1. For best results, begin by lying down on a couch or bed (or the floor) with a pillow supporting your neck. Get comfortable with a blanket or put on some cozy clothing of your choice.
2. Close your eyes and place the 2 cooled chamomile tea bags on your eyelids.
3. For even better results, place your left hand on your chest and your right hand on your lower abdomen. Practise deep belly breathing by inhaling and pushing your lower abdomen out into your hand, then exhaling and feeling the hand fall back down and the chest rise slightly. Repeat until you can feel your energy shift and know that you've taken some deep cleansing breaths.
4. After 5 to 10 minutes of applying the tea eye mask and belly breathing, remove the tea bags.
5. Apply 1 drop of serum below each eye with your ring finger. To massage it in, lightly trace your fingers in a fluid, semicircle motion, starting at the brow and moving out toward the temple and back under the eye toward the nose. Repeat as necessary.

STORAGE

Keep any extra eye serum in the fridge for refreshing results, or in a cool, dark place away from direct sunlight for up to 1 month.

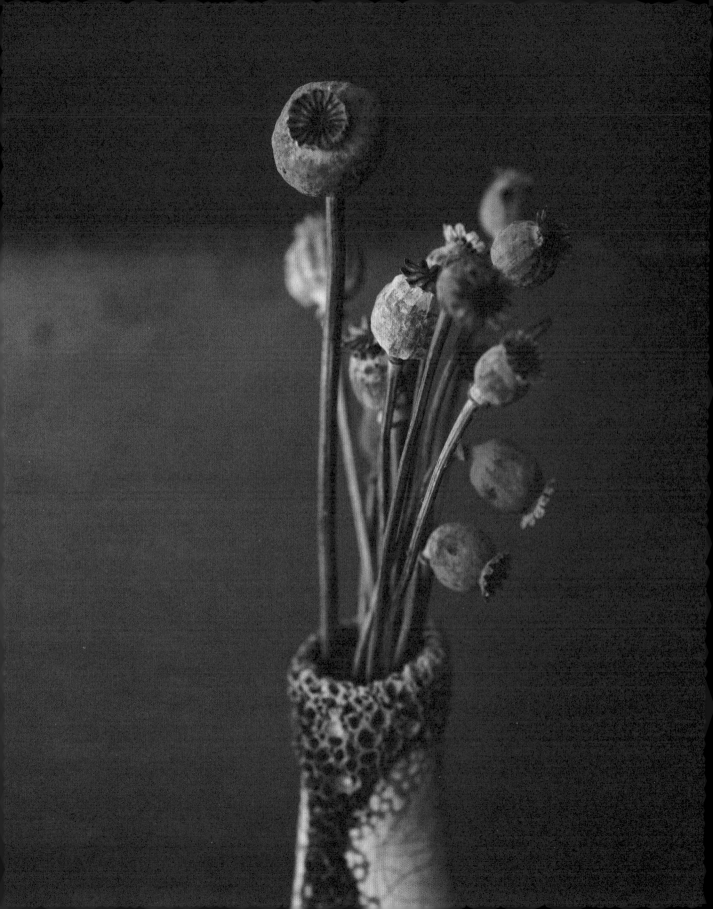

BEFORE BED FACE OILS

Taking the time to create a custom-blended moisturizing face oil might be one of the best 10-minute investments you make in your wellness routine. Having a face oil that's formulated by you is a simple way to take your self-care ritual to another level.

There's something special about putting a homemade oil on my face every evening and seeing the jar labelled with my own handwriting. Beyond feeling custom-made and thoughtful, face oils created in this form are some of the freshest and most potent you can use. By keeping the base, complex and essential oils in separate bottles, away from sunlight and air, the benefits are even stronger when you do combine them to create your custom oil.

The process of blending your own oils is very different from purchasing a pre-made evening cream or face oil at a store, which can run the risk of being affected by changes in light and temperature. There are face oils on the market with lengthy ingredient lists that can be quite expensive. This is something I don't think women should pay for. High-quality, plant-based skincare products should be affordable and readily available. Your skin deserves to drink up the goodness and nourishment from them, so you shouldn't have to pay extra for that or compromise by turning to unnatural, chemical-filled store alternatives. Happy blending, and I hope this begins the start of a very beautiful and restful bathroom apothecary in your home.

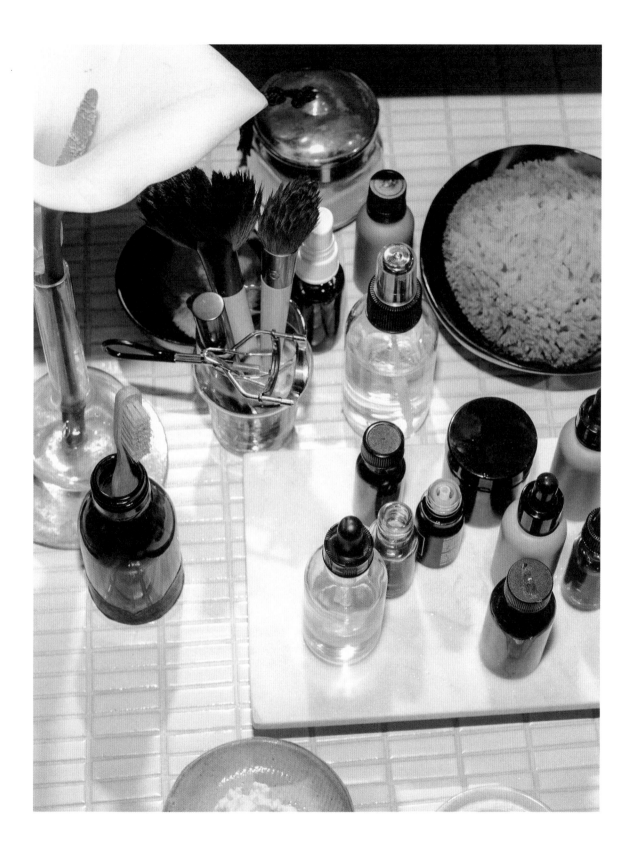

Soothing Face Oil (Sensitive Skin)

An evening face oil for gentle overnight repairing.

TIME: 5 minutes

MAKES: 2 applications

YOU'LL NEED: a 0.3-ounce (10 mL) dropper bottle or a small bowl

COMPONENTS

BASE OILS

10 drops avocado oil

5 drops apricot kernel oil

COMPLEX OILS

4 drops raspberry seed oil

4 drops blueberry seed oil

ESSENTIAL OILS

2 drops frankincense essential oil

2 drops lavender essential oil

This is my go-to face oil to calm redness and soothe and smooth the skin with its anti-inflammatory properties. This simple face oil blend is made for those with skin that is by nature more prone to redness from environmental sensitivities or inflammation from exercise, sunshine or a change in hormones. The repairing and gently rejuvenating properties of this oil make it especially lovely for those times when life is a little more stressful and your skin may be showing that.

METHOD

1. Mix the base oils, complex oils and essential oils in a dropper bottle or small bowl.
2. For best results, wait 24 hours for the components of the face oil to marry, which allows the synergy of the plant extracts to blend together in both scent and function. If you don't have time, feel free to use right away.

APPLICATION

1. Add 1 to 3 drops of face oil to the palm of your hand and rub between the hands.
2. Lightly press the hands over the face to distribute the oil.
3. Gently massage the oil into the face using the lymphatic facial massage technique (see page 135).
4. Any extra face oil can be stored for another application or rubbed on the back of your hands, neck or chest, as these are areas where extra moisture is always appreciated.

STORAGE

Keep in a cool, dark place away from direct sunlight or temperature changes in a small bowl, covered, for up to 1 week or in a dropper bottle for up to 1 month.

Replenishing Face Oil (Dry Skin)

A moisturizing face oil you can use from head to toe.

TIME: 5 minutes

MAKES: 2 applications

YOU'LL NEED: a 0.3-ounce (10 mL) dropper bottle or a small bowl

COMPONENTS

BASE OILS

10 drops avocado oil

5 drops sweet almond oil

COMPLEX OIL

5 drops pomegranate seed oil

ESSENTIAL OIL

2 drops ylang ylang essential oil

Simple and effective, this face oil is very hydrating and gentle for those times of the year when your skin may be dry or chapped due to cold and dehydrating weather. The base oils in this face oil are some of the most moisturizing you can use, and they're paired with a complex oil that improves moisture retention without being too stimulating. I chose to include only one essential oil in this blend to help with hydration, which means the final product has just a hint of aroma. This allows the slightly nutty and creamy aroma of the base oils to really shine. This simple and effective dry skin face oil will help hydrate and moisturize your skin. Feel free to use it on your hands and feet during intense dry periods.

METHOD

1. Mix the base oils, complex oil and essential oil in a dropper bottle or small bowl.
2. For best results, wait 24 hours for the components of the face oil to marry, which allows the synergy of the plant extracts to blend together in both scent and function. If you don't have time, feel free to use right away.

APPLICATION

1. Add 1 to 3 drops of face oil to the palm of your hand and rub between the hands.
2. Lightly press the hands over the face to distribute the oil.
3. Gently massage the oil into the face using the lymphatic face massage technique (see page 135).
4. Any extra face oil can be stored for another application or rubbed on the back of your hands, neck or chest, as these are areas where extra moisture is always appreciated.

STORAGE

Keep in a cool, dark place away from direct sunlight or temperature changes in a small bowl, covered, for up to 1 week or in a dropper bottle for up to 1 month.

Purifying Face Oil (Oily Skin)

A light, refreshing face oil for warm summer nights.

TIME: 5 minutes

MAKES: 2 applications

YOU'LL NEED: a 0.3-ounce (10 mL) dropper bottle or a small bowl

COMPONENTS

BASE OIL
15 drops jojoba oil

COMPLEX OILS
4 drops raspberry seed oil

3 drops sea buckthorn oil

ESSENTIAL OILS
3 drops lemon essential oil

2 drops grapefruit essential oil

Creating face oils for naturally oily skin may feel counterintuitive, but applying face oil to oily skin actually helps balance sebum production in a way that astringent face products can't. When you apply overly drying, chemical-based products, it can cue the skin to overproduce oil in response to the drying products. So, creating a hydrating face oil with naturally gentle astringent properties helps train the skin to expect moisture, without creating an abundance of shine and oil.

The jojoba oil most closely matches the natural sebum found in the skin. I chose raspberry seed oil and sea buckthorn oil as the complex oils because they're slightly astringent, which is great for preventing congestion of the pores. For the evening, I love experimenting with lemon and grapefruit essential oils because of their fresh and gentle astringent properties. They're also great to use on the face at night during warm summer months or while in more tropical climates.

METHOD

1. Mix the base oil, complex oils and essential oils in a dropper bottle or small bowl.
2. For best results, wait 24 hours for the components of the face oil to marry, which allows the synergy of the plant extracts to blend together in both scent and function. If you don't have time, feel free to use right away.

APPLICATION

1. Add 1 to 3 drops of face oil to the palm of your hand and rub between the hands.
2. Lightly press the hands over the face to distribute the oil.
3. Gently massage the oil into the face using the lymphatic face massage technique (see page 135).
4. Any extra face oil can be stored for another application or rubbed on the back of your hands, neck or chest, as these are areas where extra moisture is always appreciated.

STORAGE

Keep in a cool, dark place away from direct sunlight or temperature changes in a small bowl, covered, for up to 1 week or in a dropper bottle for up to 1 month.

Balancing Face Oil (Combination Skin)

A balanced face oil that doubles as a serum.

TIME: 5 minutes

MAKES: 2 applications

YOU'LL NEED: a 0.3-ounce (10 mL) dropper bottle or a small bowl

COMPONENTS

BASE OILS
10 drops jojoba oil

5 drops grapeseed oil

COMPLEX OILS
4 drops evening primrose oil

4 drops meadowfoam oil

ESSENTIAL OILS
3 drops lavender essential oil

2 drops sweet orange essential oil

2 drops geranium essential oil

An effective face oil for combination skin should address both the dry and the oily areas of the face while working to help the skin reach an equilibrium and balance. For this face oil, I use a combination of base oils: jojoba oil is highly moisturizing, whereas grapeseed oil is lightly moisturizing. Together, they ensure that the oil will sink into the skin at different penetration levels, which is helpful for addressing drier and oilier areas. I also include geranium essential oil because its known for its balancing properties and pair it with gentle lavender and sweet orange essential oils for a floral yet bright aroma. This evening face oil is formulated with oils that sink deeper into the skin, making it function more like a serum treatment to ensure even-looking skin.

METHOD

1. Mix the base oils, complex oils and essential oils in a dropper bottle or small bowl.
2. For best results, wait 24 hours for the components of the face oil to marry, which allows the synergy of the plant extracts to blend together in both scent and function. If you don't have time, feel free to use right away.

APPLICATION

1. Add 1 to 3 drops of face oil to the palm of your hand and rub between the hands.
2. Lightly press the hands over the face to distribute the oil.
3. Gently massage the oil into the face using the lymphatic face massage technique (see page 135).
4. Any extra face oil can be stored for another application or rubbed on the back of your hands, neck or chest, as these are areas where extra moisture is always appreciated.

STORAGE

Keep in a cool, dark place away from direct sunlight or temperature changes in a small bowl, covered, for up to 1 week or in a dropper bottle for up to 1 month.

Nourishing Face Oil (Mature Skin)

A super-hydrating face oil that smells like heaven.

TIME: 5 minutes

MAKES: 2 applications

YOU'LL NEED: a 0.3-ounce (10 mL) dropper bottle or a small bowl

COMPONENTS

BASE OILS

10 drops apricot kernel oil

5 drops plum oil

COMPLEX OILS

4 drops rosehip oil

4 drops meadowfoam oil

ESSENTIAL OILS

3 drops cedarwood essential oil

3 drops rosemary essential oil

2 drops ylang ylang essential oil

For mature skin, I love creating dynamic and recharging face oils. I use rich essential oils and complex oils that feel deeply hydrating and have a deep and complex aroma. The emphasis of this oil is on antioxidant and cell-repairing complex oils, like rosehip and meadowfoam oils. I then pair those with moisturizing base oils like apricot kernel oil and plum oil to make the skin feel full and soft. The essential oils in this face oil are some of the most potent, in both aroma and properties. A high-quality ylang ylang oil is almost sap-like and very calming to the skin, while cedarwood and rosemary stimulate circulation to the surface of the skin (albeit gently), thus promoting repair and cell turnover. I love using this face oil after a good mask and exfoliation.

METHOD

1. Mix the base oils, complex oils and essential oils in a dropper bottle or small bowl.
2. For best results, wait 24 hours for the components of the face oil to marry, which allows the synergy of the plant extracts to blend together in both scent and function. If you don't have time, feel free to use right away.

APPLICATION

1. Add 1 to 3 drops of face oil to the palm of your hand and rub between the hands.
2. Lightly press the hands over the face to distribute the oil.
3. Gently massage the oil into the face using the lymphatic face massage technique (see page 135).
4. Any extra face oil can be stored for another application or rubbed on the back of your hands, neck or chest, as these are areas where extra moisture is always appreciated.

STORAGE

Keep in a cool, dark place away from direct sunlight or temperature changes in a small bowl, covered, for up to 1 week or in a dropper bottle for up to 1 month.

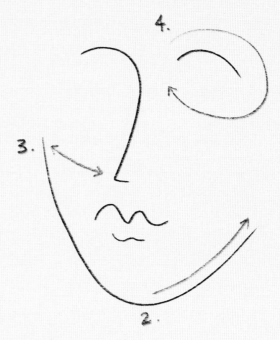

LYMPHATIC FACIAL MASSAGE

A simple lymphatic facial massage is an easy way to turn your daily cleansing and moisturizing routine into a spa ritual. This technique helps improve circulation and blood flow to the skin and, in doing so, increases blood flow and helps naturally promote healthy lymph drainage from the face. It targets tension points in the face, which helps relax muscles and improves your ability to produce more collagen in the face.

STEPS

1. Using your fingers, massage a thin layer of face oil on the face.
2. Starting at the chin, massage the skin from the chin outward along the jawline to the base of the ear. Repeat, alternating sides.
3. From the side of the nose, alternate massaging from the nose, along the cheekbone, to the ear.
4. Starting at the inner edge of the brow, follow the brow line to the outer edge of the brow. Then, move below the eye and along the top of the cheekbone, finishing in the inner corner of the eye.
5. Repeat these steps on both sides of the face while breathing deeply.

LAST STEP LIP TREATMENTS

The health and hydration of the lips and the area around the lips is often taken for granted until further into the aging process. The products we use on our lips and how we take care of the skin around our lips is something I don't take lightly. It's not about being anti-aging—I am very happy about the aging process and the wisdom that living a long, full life brings. For me, it's about taking care of the lips and the area around them, and hydrating them is a way to take a moment to yourself throughout the day.

I hope you enjoy these nourishing lip treatments and recognize that they are just one of the many ways you take care of your beauty, along with speaking words of kindness, taking time for yourself and nourishing your body and skin with whole, natural, plant-based products.

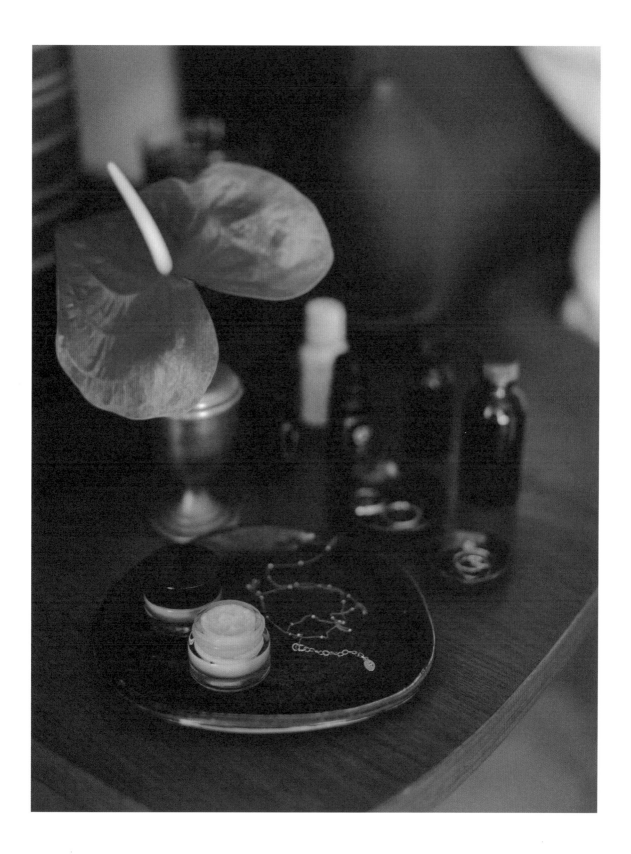

Nourishing Brown Sugar and Honey Lip Scrub

A luxurious lip scrub for pillow-soft lips.

TIME: 3 minutes

MAKES: 5 lip scrub treatments

YOU'LL NEED: a small bowl and a 1-ounce (30 mL) glass jar with a lid

COMPONENTS

1 tablespoon organic brown sugar

1 teaspoon organic liquid honey (or add until a paste forms with the brown sugar)

1 drop organic pure vanilla extract

1 drop sweet orange essential oil

This is a simple step to add to your evening routine. I love doing a lip scrub a few times a week right before brushing my teeth. Depending on the season, sometimes I'll switch up the essential oil in the recipe, replacing the sweet orange essential oil with peppermint essential oil in the summer for something light and fresh. For this year-round recipe, I love the vanilla and honey mixed with the sweet orange essential oil for a sweet yet fresh aroma.

METHOD

1. In a small bowl, add the brown sugar and honey and stir with a metal spoon to combine (wooden spoons stick to the honey too much).
2. Add the vanilla and sweet orange essential oil and mix thoroughly.

APPLICATION

1. Using your finger, apply ½ teaspoon of the lip scrub to the lips.
2. Rub the lip scrub into the lips and exfoliate gently.
3. Let the paste sit on the lips for at least 1 minute or while you do the rest of your face cleansing and moisturizing routine. Rinse off with warm water.
4. Apply the Healing and Hydrating Lip Balm (page 139) afterwards to hydrate the lips before sleeping.

STORAGE

Keep in a cool, dry place away from direct sunlight for up to 2 months.

Healing and Hydrating Lip Balm

An ultra-nourishing lip balm that lives on your nightstand.

TIME: 20 minutes

MAKES: 0.67 ounce (20 mL) lip balm

YOU'LL NEED: a 1-ounce (30 mL) glass jar with a lid

COMPONENTS

½ teaspoon organic grated beeswax

½ teaspoon organic shea butter

½ teaspoon jojoba oil

½ teaspoon hemp seed oil

2 drops rosemary essential oil

2 drops lavender essential oil

10 drops vitamin E 1000 IU (squeezed from vitamin E capsules or liquid serum vitamin E; optional)

The final step in my evening routine is a healing and hydrating lip balm. I like this one because the scent and feeling of it has now become one of the last steps in my bedtime ritual. It's an especially important part of my routine during the winter months or while travelling in dry climates. I make this balm in small batches and keep it in a little jar beside my bed—each jar usually lasts 2 months. The essential oils used in this balm are meant to be relaxing and rejuvenating, and I chose them to have a centring and grounding aroma yet be nourishing and hydrating for the skin of the lips. When applying this balm, also apply some to the skin surrounding the lips, as it helps with keeping the lip area feeling plump and full.

METHOD

1. Using a double boiler, melt the beeswax, shea butter, jojoba oil and hemp seed oil and stir to combine.
2. Remove from the heat. When the mixture starts to cool, about 5 minutes, you'll see the colour start to turn milky.
3. When the liquid is milky but not yet firm, add the rosemary and lavender essential oils and vitamin E (if using). Stir to combine and then pour into the glass jar.
4. Allow to cool completely, uncovered, until the moisture has evaporated and the balm is in a solid state.

APPLICATION

1. Using your finger, apply the lip balm to the lips and surrounding area before bed or whenever you need hydration.

STORAGE

Keep in a cool, dry place away from direct sunlight for up to 2 months.

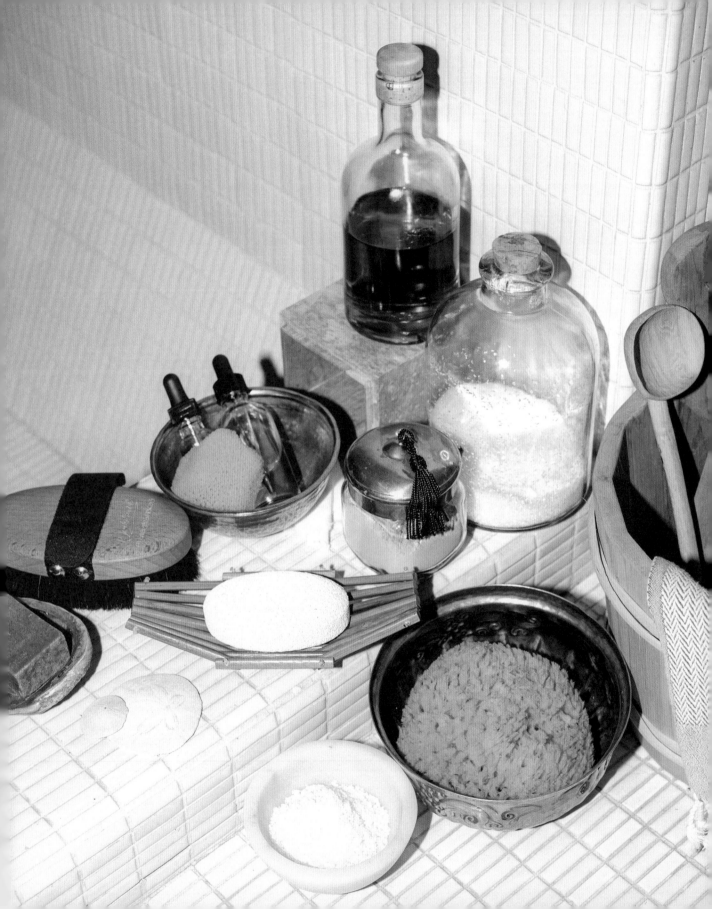

BODY

If you're anything like me, you live a lot in your own head—thinking, overanalyzing, dreaming and hypothesizing. It wasn't until a few years ago that I began to consciously connect with my body. I started creating rituals and habits that reminded me to breathe, ground my feet and connect to an energy outside of the business in my head. This section of the book focuses on some of the techniques I've learned from teachers and masters of energy, as well as a few of my own creations that use aroma to cue the brain to reconnect with the physical body.

The dynamic of combining aroma, touch and breath is powerful. Simple daily rituals that scrub and cleanse the body have helped me coach my mind to shed and let go of any heaviness from the day. Too often we only "connect" with our body through exercise (if we're able to fit in a workout), but that connection can be superficial and usually performance-based. We also connect with our bodies while we put our clothes on and assess how they fit, or when we stand in front of a mirror or towel off after a shower. It's far too easy to take that time to judge and critique ourselves. By carving out quick moments to nurture and take care of the incredible body that helps you experience and make moves in this world, you're doing both your mind and your body a huge favour. Making these connections can be simple—whether it's a foot soak after standing for 8 hours at work, a body scrub to remind yourself that there is always an opportunity for a fresh start or a quick hand massage before bed. It has been shown that when women carve out just 10 minutes for themselves, they show up with more energy, perspective and clarity for the next 24 hours. That's pretty amazing.

The awareness and consciousness I've gained through integrating the following habits has been incredibly transformative for me. I credit many of these practices with enabling me to be a more grounded leader, a more present partner and a more aware friend. I truly hope you find time to try these practices and to experiment and personalize them in whichever ways serve you best.

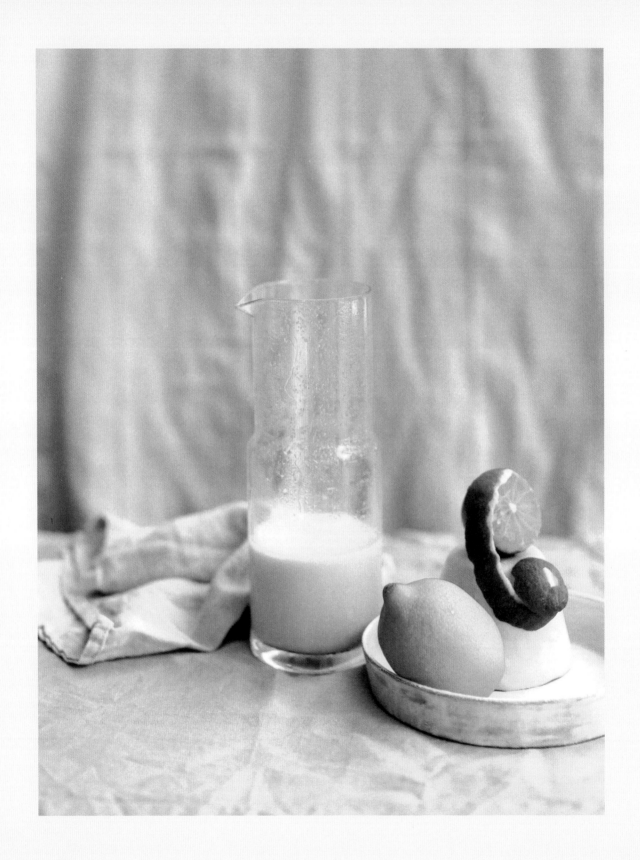

MORNING BODY RITUALS

It truly surprises me how much you can fit into a morning if you're creative and intentional about it. I used to scurry from bed to laptop to shower to closet to bag to key to door. Now, my pattern looks similar, but there are a few hidden practices and spa moments woven in between. These morning rituals help me feel that I've front-loaded my day for myself and my wellness (even if no one else at home would realize it). The morning is a time when you can set the pace and energy for the day. A shift in how you show up can happen if you take just a little time for yourself before taking on the world. This section contains a few of my favourite ways to start the morning. I'm not suggesting you fit them all in, but experiment each week and choose a few to try with the intention of finding some rituals that might become a more permanent part of your morning routine. Happy creating and good morning, beautiful.

SHOWER SPA MOMENTS

I love turning a quick morning shower into a full-on spa experience. Among the morning chaos of alarms going off, inbox alerts popping up or children calling you—no one will know you've created a little oasis in the shower (even if for only 3 minutes). Here are my favourite shower rituals that incorporate aroma as a way to help cue the brain and body to wake up and function in a more alert and engaged state.

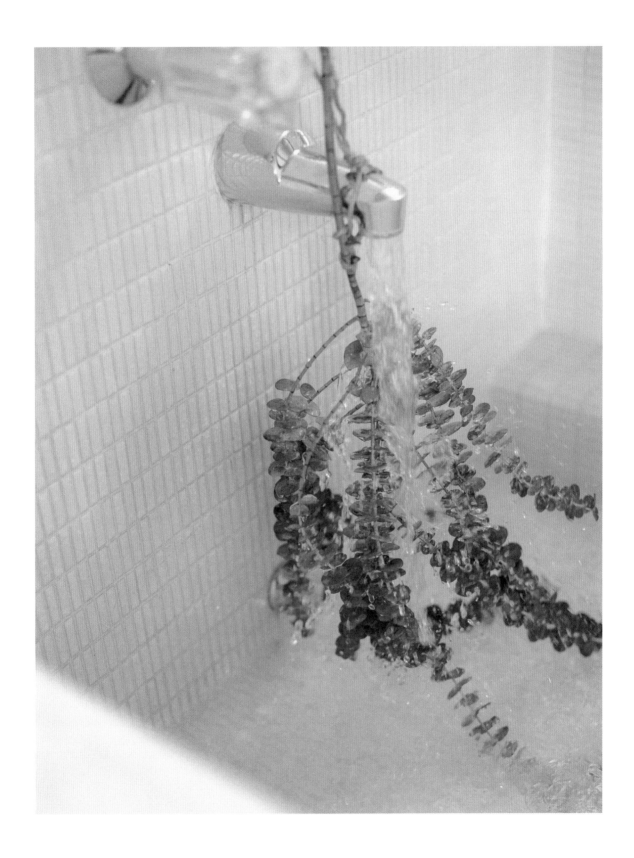

Eucalyptus Steam Shower

A few glorious minutes to yourself.

TIME: 1 minute

MAKES: 1 eucalyptus steam shower

COMPONENTS

3 to 5 drops eucalyptus essential oil

This steam shower is for those mornings when you need an extra pick-me-up and a reminder to take a deep breath (or for every morning, really). Creating a quick eucalyptus steam is the perfect practice to awaken your senses gently and invigorate your respiratory system. And yes, it truly is the easiest and most cost-effective spa experience you'll ever have.

I ensure that I make this part of my morning routine during cold and flu season. The benefits of the eucalyptus essential oil are refreshing to the nose and throat. The heat from the shower water helps the volatile oils in the eucalyptus essential oil to vaporize, which allows the antimicrobial, antiseptic and anti-inflammatory properties of the oil to fill the shower. It's a really simple and healthy way to start your day during a time of year when it can be especially hard to keep your wellness on track.

METHOD AND APPLICATION

1. Prepare a comfortable, hot shower (you'll want it hot enough so the shower area has some steam).
2. While in the shower, apply the eucalyptus essential oil to the palm of your hand and rub your hands together briskly. Cup your hands and bring them close to your face. Breathe deeply.
3. Rinse the oil off your hands with the shower water.

Full Body Detox Steam

An invigorating steam that wakes up your entire body.

TIME: 3 minutes

MAKES: 1 full body detox steam

YOU'LL NEED: 1 hand towel

COMPONENTS

15 to 20 drops of your favourite
essential oils

This is a simple and super-invigorating way to feel a deep and intense cleanse of the skin, while fully enjoying the natural benefits of essential oils. I love using grapefruit, lemongrass and eucalyptus essential oils in this detox steam because the hot water intensifies the aromas and I instantly feel refreshed and more awake. Full body steams are also a great way to experience the topical benefits of some of your favourite essential oils. For this detox steam, you really only need two things: your favourite essential oils and a large face cloth or hand towel to bring into the shower with you.

METHOD

1. Prepare a comfortable, hot shower (you'll want it hot enough so the shower area has some steam).
2. While in the shower, wet a hand towel with the hot shower water, then ring out excess water.
3. Apply the essential oils to the towel.

APPLICATION

1. Wrap the towel around the back of your neck and your shoulders, then turn your back toward the shower.
2. Allow the heat of the shower and shower water to hit the towel.
3. Stand still and take 3 deep belly breaths. Breathe in through the nose, pause, exhale through the mouth, pause. Repeat 2 more times.
4. After the deep breaths, ring out the towel and use it to scrub the body, moving upward from the feet toward the shoulders in small circular motions.

STORAGE

Wash the towel afterwards or allow it to hang-dry for the next use. Keep your favourite essential oils in the shower to make them accessible for future detox steams.

SHOWER FIZZES

A unique way to add scent to your morning shower routine is with a shower fizz. Making them is a great weekend project, and the explosion of scented oils and invigorating fizz is an easy way to make your morning shower routine a little more upbeat. I find it brings a much-needed lightness to stressful mornings. I've often used them on mornings when I have an important meeting or an intense day lined up. I'm all about sneaking simple moments of playfulness into the everyday routine.

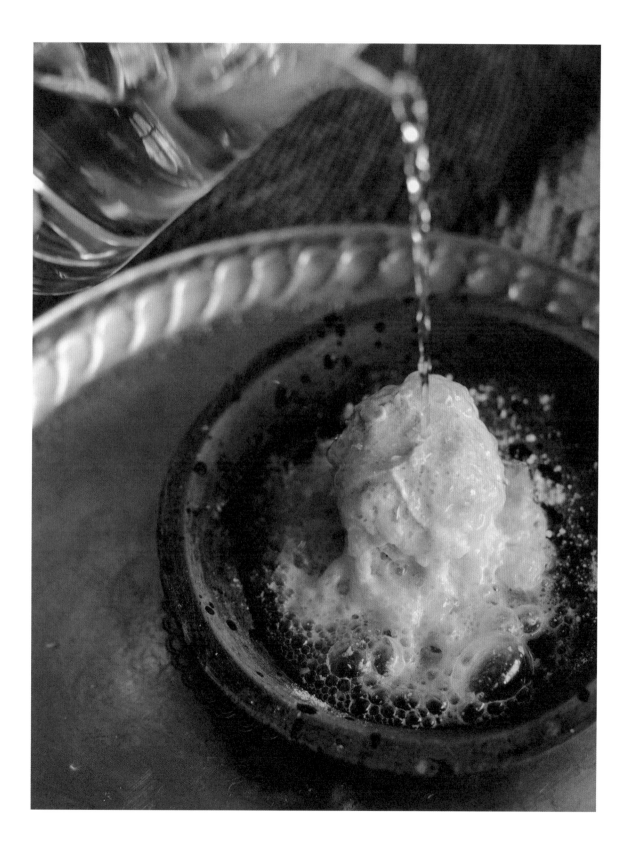

Fresh Start Shower Fizz

An uplifting fizz that makes your morning shower a little more fun.

TIME: 30 minutes + overnight to cure

MAKES: 16 fizz cubes

YOU'LL NEED: a medium bowl, a flexible ice cube tray and an airtight container with a lid

COMPONENTS

1 cup baking soda

½ cup citric acid

½ cup cornstarch

1 teaspoon water

3 teaspoons sweet almond oil

30 drops sweet orange essential oil

15 drops peppermint essential oil

For this shower fizz, I love using sweet orange and peppermint essential oils. The sweet citrus of the orange feels rejuvenating and smells like freshly squeezed orange juice (does anything else smell more quintessentially like morning?), and the peppermint instantly makes me feel fresh, clean and awake. It's a favourite to use during the summer months because it helps me start the day feeling uplifted.

METHOD

1. In a medium bowl, combine the baking soda, citric acid and cornstarch.
2. Slowly add the water and the oils and mix together until a wet sand consistency is achieved.
3. Lightly pack the mixture into the compartments of an ice cube tray (I love using ones with cute shapes).
4. Leave the mixture to cure overnight in a dry space away from temperature changes and sunlight.
5. Carefully remove the fizz cubes from the tray and allow them to dry further on a towel for 2 to 4 hours, depending on how humid your climate is.

APPLICATION

1. Place 2 fizz cubes on the floor of your shower where water will splash onto them (just make sure they are not getting hit directly with a constant stream of water).
2. Let the water splash onto the cubes and allow them to fizz.
3. Take some deep breaths as the aroma releases and stretch your arms upward, helping to open the lungs and improve deep breathing.

STORAGE

Keep in an airtight container in a cool, dry place for up to 1 month.

Solid to the Earth Shower Fizz

A grounding fizz that channels outdoor shower vibes.

TIME: 30 minutes + overnight to cure

MAKES: 16 fizz cubes

YOU'LL NEED: a medium bowl, a small bowl, a flexible ice cube tray and an airtight container with a lid

COMPONENTS

1 cup baking soda

½ cup citric acid

½ cup Epsom salts

3 teaspoons sweet almond oil

20 drops bergamot essential oil

20 drops cedarwood essential oil

10 drops spruce essential oil

This is one of my favourite ways to set the tone for the morning. The fun fizz paired with the grounding and invigorating aromas of cedarwood, spruce and bergamot essential oils helps me wake up naturally and set my intentions for the day. I suggest using this fizz on cozy winter mornings or when you want to feel a little closer to nature but the only place you're going is to the office. Getting a nature fix in the shower isn't the same as "forest bathing," but in a city apartment or suburban neighbourhood, it's a great (and more realistic) alternative.

METHOD

1. In a medium bowl, combine the baking soda, citric acid and Epsom salts.
2. In a small bowl, mix together the oils.
3. Slowy add the essential oil mixture, 1 spoonful at a time, and the water to the baking soda mixture. Mix together until a wet sand consistency is achieved.
4. Lightly pack the mixture into the compartments of the ice cube tray.
5. Leave the mixture to cure overnight in a dry space away from temperature changes and sunlight.
6. Carefully remove the fizz cubes from the tray and allow them to dry further on a towel for 2 to 4 hours, depending on how humid your climate is.

APPLICATION

1. Place 2 fizz cubes on the floor of your shower where water will splash onto them (just make sure they are not getting hit directly with a constant stream of water).
2. Let the water splash onto the cubes and allow them to fizz.
3. Take some deep breaths as the aroma releases and stretch your arms upward, helping to open the lungs and improve deep breathing.

STORAGE

Keep in an airtight container in a cool, dry place for up to 1 month.

INVIGORATING BODY SCRUBS

Body scrubs are something I love starting my morning with because they make me feel fresh and ready for a new day. It's a simple way to turn your morning routine into a spa experience, and they're easy to make in batches so you can always have some on hand. Feel free to make any of these recipes in double or triple batches and keep them in airtight jars in your shower, but try not to let water get into the jars. The possibilities are endless for homemade body scrubs; I love to mix up the essential oils and exfoliating ingredients I use seasonally—sugar and citrus in the summer and nourishing, rich coconut oils and oats in the winter. I hope the recipes and practices I have created inspire you to make and mix your own.

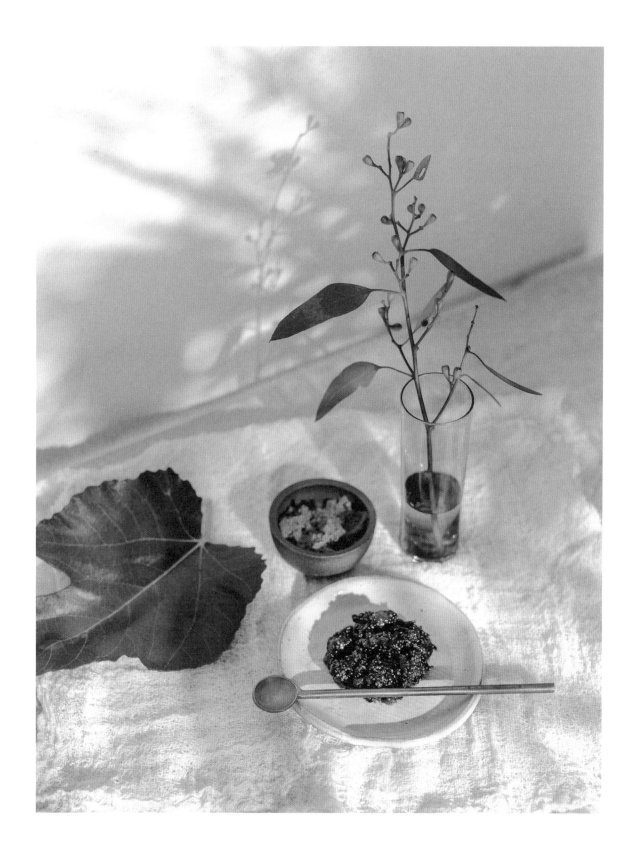

Coffee and Bergamot Scrub

A stimulating body scrub that instantly leaves you feeling more awake.

TIME: 10 minutes

MAKES: ½ cup body scrub, enough for 1 to 2 full body treatments

YOU'LL NEED: a small bowl, a spoon and an airtight container with a lid

COMPONENTS

¼ cup coffee grinds

2 tablespoons organic brown sugar

2 tablespoons organic solid virgin coconut oil

10 drops bergamot essential oil

Coffee is an essential part of my life. In all seriousness, my dad got me into espresso at a relatively young age and gave me a taste and love for good-quality espresso in a way that makes it a necessary part of my morning. Beyond helping my day start off right, coffee makes winter days warm, is an excuse to get together with friends and, in quiet moments, provides motivation to get a task done or a project finished with each sip.

I created this coffee body scrub as a way to live more environmentally friendly, as I wanted to do something with the coffee grinds I was left with each morning. Living in the city, it's harder to compost them like my parents do back in their rural country home.

So, wanting to recycle and re-use as many things in my home as I can, I decided to use the grounds each day in a morning body scrub. It turned out to be a great way to start my mornings and a nice way to re-use things. The aroma of the grounds helps me wake up even more, and the caffeine topically helps stimulate circulation and also improves alertness.

METHOD

1. Combine all components in a small bowl. Mix with a spoon until evenly combined and the mixture forms a paste.
2. Place in an airtight container and keep in your shower.
3. Breathe deeply.

APPLICATION

1. Starting at the feet, apply the scrub with your hands in small circular motions over the whole body.
2. Once completely covered in the scrub, rinse it off in the shower.

STORAGE

Keep in an airtight container and try to avoid water getting into the scrub. The scrub should keep for up to 2 weeks if kept away from moisture.

Cozy Citrus Sugar and Oatmeal Scrub

An invigorating body scrub that warms you up from head to toe.

TIME: 5 minutes

MAKES: 1½ cups body scrub, enough for 3 to 4 full body treatments

YOU'LL NEED: a medium bowl, a spoon and an airtight container with a lid

COMPONENTS

½ cup quick oats

½ cup organic brown sugar

½ cup organic solid virgin coconut oil

10 drops sweet orange essential oil

10 drops grapefruit essential oil

10 drops tea tree essential oil

Whether it's sweater weather or beach time, this easy everyday sugar oatmeal scrub is perfect for combination skin or a combination of seasons. The oatmeal and coconut oil add moisture to the skin, while the sugar exfoliates and the grapefruit, tea tree and sweet orange essential oils leave your body smelling fresh and feeling cleansed. The essential oils chosen for this scrub provide a fresh and invigorating morning aroma and contain natural antimicrobial properties that help with truly cleansing the skin. Consider it the perfect morning shower ritual—because your skin should feel soft and cleansed every day of the week, and clean doesn't need to mean stripped of its natural oils.

METHOD

1. In a medium bowl, mix together the quick oats, sugar and coconut oil.
2. Add the essential oils and mix together with a spoon (or your hands) until fully incorporated.

APPLICATION

1. Starting at the feet, apply the scrub with your hands in small circular motions over the whole body.
2. Once completely covered in the scrub, rinse it off in the shower.
3. Breathe deeply.

STORAGE

Keep in an airtight container and try to avoid water getting into the scrub. The scrub should keep for up to 2 weeks if kept away from moisture.

Fig and Eucalyptus Scrub

A decadent yet super-simple body scrub for pampering yourself.

TIME: 30 minutes

MAKES: 3 ounces (90 mL) scrub

YOU'LL NEED: a small bowl, a fork, a saucepan, a wooden spoon and a glass jar with a lid

COMPONENTS

2 large ripe figs (or 4 dried figs soaked overnight in water to rehydrate)

1 tablespoon organic solid virgin coconut oil

1 tablespoon sweet almond oil

4 tablespoons organic brown sugar

2 drops eucalyptus essential oil

Figs have always felt like a luxurious, indulgent fruit to me. Best used in a salad or on a summer platter, I love that they are particular in terms of when they can be eaten and that without the correct ripeness, eating them just isn't the same experience. I first tried using figs in my homemade body products when I had some left over after making a summer salad and read that their seeds make a great exfoliant. The seeds really are a gentle exfoliant provided by Mother Nature that leaves your skin feeling dessert-like and nourished in a way that only a whole fruit can. The brown sugar in this recipe provides another method of exfoliating and adds to the luxurious aroma and feeling on the skin.

METHOD

1. Peel the ripe figs and mash with a fork in a small bowl until they turn to mush (or purée in a blender or food processor).
2. Add the figs, coconut oil and sweet almond oil to a saucepan and stir together until melted and combined. Remove from heat.
3. When the mixture begins to cool, add the brown sugar and eucalyptus essential oil.
4. Pour the mixture into a glass jar and let cool fully before putting the lid on top.

APPLICATION

1. Starting at the feet, apply the scrub with your hands in small circular motions over the whole body.
2. Once completely covered in the scrub, rinse it off in the shower.
3. Breathe deeply.

STORAGE

Keep in an airtight container and try to avoid water getting into the scrub. The scrub should keep for up to 1 week if kept away from moisture. Store in the fridge for best results.

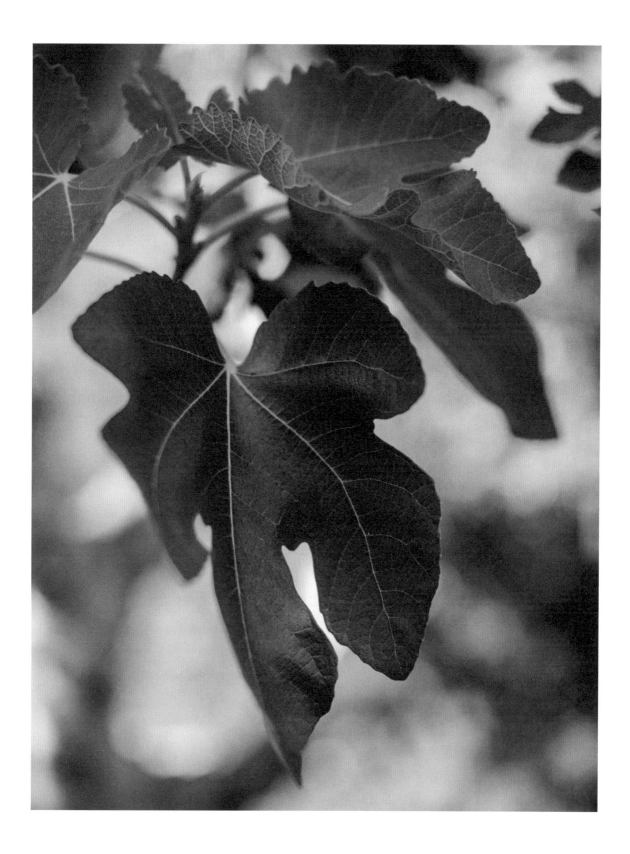

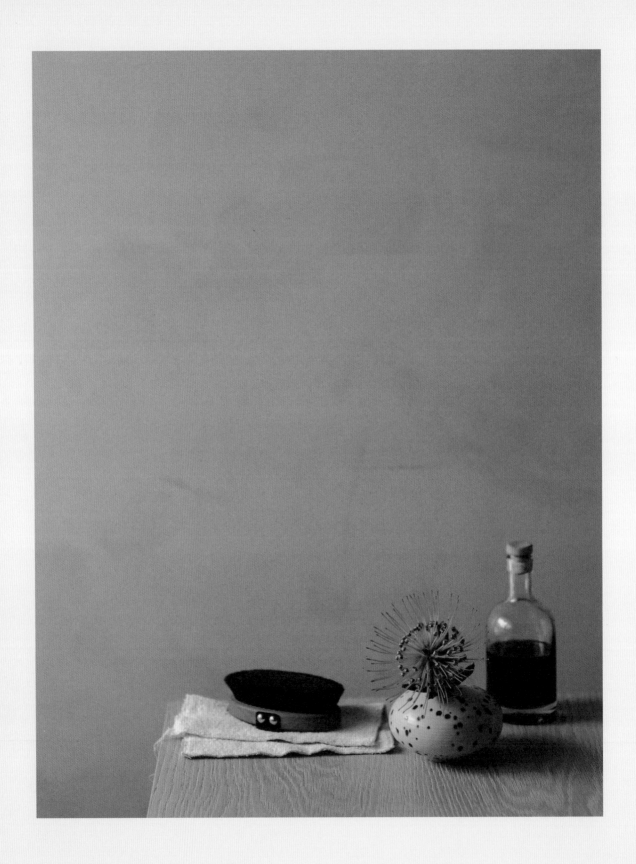

DRY BRUSHING

Brushing the skin is a practice that has been recorded in cultures dating back hundreds of years in Japan and ancient Greece. It's a simple ritual of exfoliating the skin with a dry, natural bristle brush that provides both internal and external benefits to the body and skin.

Beyond exfoliating and eliminating dead skin cells, dry brushing also helps unblock hair follicles, leaving you with smooth, soft skin that has a natural glow. The pressure and direction of brushing also stimulates and mimics the direction of your body's natural lymphatic drainage patterns. By applying and increasing circulation, dry brushing stimulates the skin while keeping the skin pores clear, so that the body can perspire freely.

It can take a few attempts to get used to and enjoy the feeling of the bristles during dry brushing. Once integrated into your wellness routine two to three times a week, it will become something you look forward to. For me, it's a practice that I enjoy, and it often reminds me to think about what else I want to purge or get rid of. Getting rid of the layer of skin that no longer serves you is a great time to reflect on the thoughts and emotional patterns that might also not be benefiting you.

This ritual should take just 3 to 7 minutes, depending on how much time you have. It's recommended to do it in the morning because it helps increase circulation and can improve energy; however, I enjoy dry brushing before bathing in the evenings. I find it's a nice way to sink into reflection, and I like ending my day with the fresh feeling I get from it, both physically and mentally.

TECHNIQUE
1. Brushing should be performed on dry skin.
2. Always ensure that you brush in a direction toward the heart.
3. Apply enough pressure to stimulate the skin but never so much that the bristles are scratching you.

PATTERN
1. Start at your feet and brush upward toward the heart using small upward strokes.
2. For the arms, start at the hands and work upward toward the shoulders.
3. For the torso and stomach, ensure that you work in a counterclockwise pattern toward the heart.

OIL BODY WASHES

I love using oil-based body washes because they leave my skin feeling squeaky-clean but not stripped of its natural oils and moisture. In the past, I've found that drugstore body washes tend to be full of toxic chemicals and foaming agents that aren't natural, while the natural alternatives often have uninspired aromas. That's why I love making my own body washes and soap products. I first became passionate about this while travelling in Morocco. The spa culture (traditionally known as hammam) is a bath house where you are covered in black soap, then scrubbed and steamed from head to toe. The hammam experience in Morocco introduced me to the beauty and simplicity of a well-made soap. It showed me that a spa experience doesn't need to be considered a luxury—soap, scrubbing and exfoliating at a community bath house are very much a normal part of the week. I have since created a number of signature soap products inspired by my time in Morocco, combined with my own modern take on aroma. I hope these simple and natural body washes add some exotic spa vibes to your morning routine.

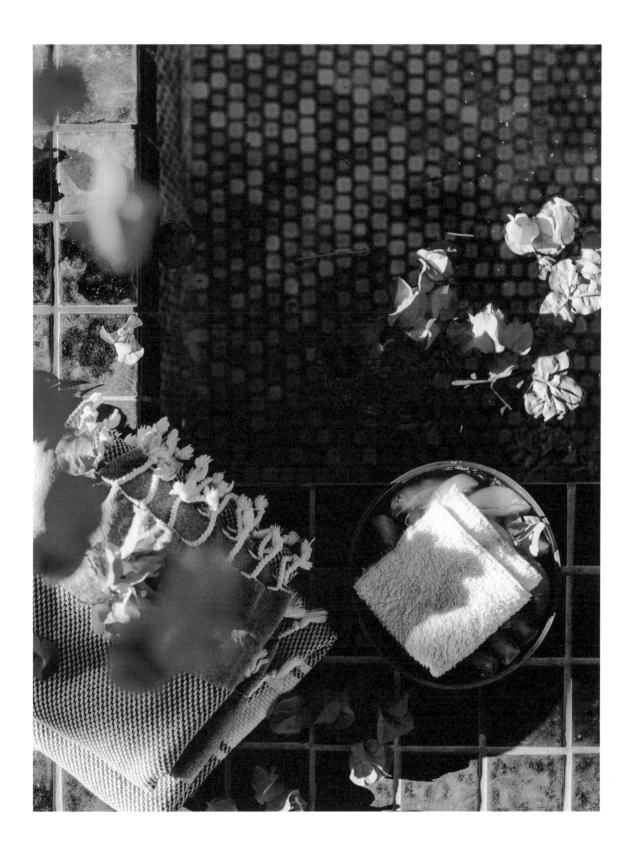

Fountain Flowers Body Wash

A body wash that captures the soft yet energizing energy of Morocco.

TIME: 3 minutes

MAKES: 9.47 ounces (280 mL) body wash

YOU'LL NEED: a medium bowl and a 12-ounce (360 mL) bottle with a pump top

COMPONENTS

⅔ cup unscented liquid Castile soap

⅓ cup organic liquid honey

2 tablespoons base oil (jojoba, sweet almond or grapeseed)

20 drops geranium essential oil

20 drops cedarwood essential oil

10 drops frankincense essential oil

10 drops ylang ylang essential oil

This body wash is inspired by a photograph I took of flower petals in a Moroccan fountain on an old clay wall. I had just finished a session at a spa that locals in Marrakech go to on a daily or weekly basis. The foundation was old and covered in ceramic tiles, but the water was crisp and clear, and the flower petals were a beautiful bold pink. It's an image that has stuck in my head because it fully embodies the exotic and fresh yet beautifully worn-in energy and aesthetic of Morocco.

This body wash has a flower-forward aroma, as a nod to Morocco's love of roses and florals, along with a smokiness inspired by incense and the country's spa rituals. I've included cedarwood and frankincense to give complexity to the soap's aroma—one that you won't find in a store. This body wash is made with a liquid Castile soap to ensure that it has enough suds, without the addition of any chemical foaming agents. It's always nice to have some bubbles in your soap, but never at the expense of using chemicals. I hope this product creates a Moroccan oasis in your morning shower, like it still does for me.

METHOD

1. Add all components to a medium bowl or directly into a bottle with a pump top.
2. Stir or shake gently to combine.

APPLICATION

1. Shake gently before each use.
2. To use, place 1 to 3 teaspoons on a natural face cloth or directly on the body and rub into the skin to create a foaming, sudsy wash.
3. Remember to breathe, take in the scent and then rinse off.

STORAGE

Keep in a bottle with a lid in your shower or bathroom for up to 6 months. Avoid moisture and water coming in direct contact with the body wash for a long shelf life.

Morning Mint Tea Body Wash

A body wash inspired by mint tea and a tranquil Moroccan morning.

TIME: 3 minutes

MAKES: 9.47 ounces (280 mL) body wash

YOU'LL NEED: a medium bowl and a 12-ounce (360 mL) bottle with a pump top

COMPONENTS

⅔ cup unscented liquid Castile soap

⅓ cup organic liquid honey

2 tablespoons base oil (jojoba, sweet almond or grapeseed)

20 drops peppermint essential oil

10 drops rosemary essential oil

10 drops lemon essential oil

This body wash was also inspired by my travels in Morocco—this time by the mint tea I fell in love with. The tea is made with green tea and fresh mint leaves, then sugar and honey are added to the boiling water as it all brews. The result is an incredibly sweet yet fresh aroma and taste that I wanted to recreate in a body wash. It seemed fitting to incorporate this into a morning body ritual because the mint tea in Morocco is something you start your day with in the market before adventuring.

To recreate one of my favourite Moroccan rituals, I used peppermint essential oil to give the aroma of the fresh mint in the tea and combined it with rosemary essential oil to give the herbal quality of the green tea. Finally, organic liquid honey is included in this recipe as a special component because it helps the soap become smooth and nourishing and adds a sweetness to the aroma, much like that of the tea.

This is my go-to everyday body wash, and it also makes a lovely wash for after a morning workout. I hope that if you don't get to try Moroccan mint tea, you at least can experience its freshness re-created in this body wash.

METHOD

1. Add all components to a medium bowl or directly into a bottle with a pump top.
2. Stir or shake gently to combine.

APPLICATION

1. Shake gently before each use.
2. To use, place 1 to 3 teaspoons on a natural face cloth or directly on the body and rub into the skin to create a foaming, sudsy wash.
3. Remember to breathe, take in the scent and then rinse off.

STORAGE

Keep in a bottle with a lid in your shower or bathroom for up to 6 months. Avoid moisture and water coming in direct contact with the body wash for a long shelf life.

NATURAL SHAMPOO

Making your own hair products for the shower may seem daunting, but in all honesty, the products we use on our hair have become incredibly overcomplicated. These formulations often leave us with more additives, preservatives and chemicals (and synthetic aromas) in our hair than actual nourishing components. Depending on your hair type, switching to natural shampoo and conditioner can be a slow process—try mixing 1 teaspoon at a time into your regular hair products and showering with those. After a few tries, you can slowly transition to a natural shampoo and conditioner, and you should find that your hair and scalp become even better at regulating their own oil production and moisture level. The following recipe has been my go-to natural shampoo. Knowing that the products I put directly on my head are completely free of chemicals and preservatives is a lifestyle change I'm incredibly proud of.

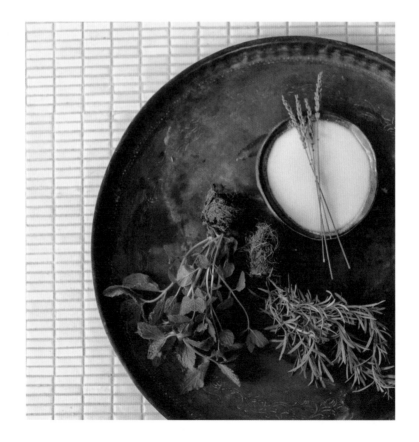

Rosemary Calming and Clarifying Shampoo

A homemade shampoo that proves once you go natural, you'll never go back.

TIME: 5 minutes

MAKES: 4 ounces (120 mL) shampoo

YOU'LL NEED: a 4-ounce (120 mL) bottle with a pump top

COMPONENTS

¼ cup organic canned full-fat coconut milk

¼ cup unscented liquid Castile soap

20 drops rosemary essential oil

10 drops lavender essential oil

5 drops peppermint essential oil

1 teaspoon jojoba oil or sweet almond oil (optional, if you have extra-dry hair)

This clarifying shampoo is designed to promote scalp health just as much as hair health. The aroma of this product reminds me of an outdoor spa I visited on the west coast of Canada. They made their own bath products, and while using the shampoo in the outdoor pools, I was reminded that there are more simple ways of living. Eventually, after using more natural products, my hair became accustomed to a lower sudsing shampoo. My scalp also came to crave time with the shampoo and felt more hydrated and clean than when I used traditional shampoos.

The essential oils in this shampoo were chosen for scalp health and will result in a slightly tingling sensation as they help clean and stimulate the hair follicles and hair shafts at the base of the scalp. This tingling sensation is a nice addition to your morning shower routine, and the coconut milk has a cooling effect that makes this shampoo extremely lovely in summer months or while on vacation.

I also love using this shampoo as a shaving cream. The coconut milk smooths out any razor burn, and the essential oils help stimulate and prevent bacteria in the hair shafts, making for an ultra-clean shave.

METHOD

1. Add all components to a bottle with a pump top.
2. Shake gently to combine until the coconut milk is blended in and the mixture has a smooth consistency.

APPLICATION

1. Shake gently before each use.
2. Pump 1 to 3 teaspoons of shampoo into the palm of your hand (or as much as your hair needs that day).
3. Apply to hair and massage into the scalp with fingers. Add more shampoo as needed.
4. Rinse from the hair.
5. Follow with hair tonic and conditioner, if desired.

STORAGE

Keep in an airtight container or a bottle with a lid in a cool, dry place or in your shower for up to 1 week. Avoid moisture and water coming in direct contact with the shampoo for a long shelf life.

HAIR TONICS

Hair tonics are not used often in home hair treatments, but they're a regular step in salons to help tone the colour and texture of the hair. Made with simple ingredients, these tonics are designed to provide a lightweight and colour-boosting addition to your morning routine. Plus, they're easy to make in large batches to use throughout the week. I especially love using hair tonics after a workout or when my hair and scalp feel extra sensitive after a long run. The components of each of these tonics are designed for a specific hair type, but remember that the needs of your hair change with the seasons and activities you do, so feel free to experiment with other recipes and venture outside your "hair type."

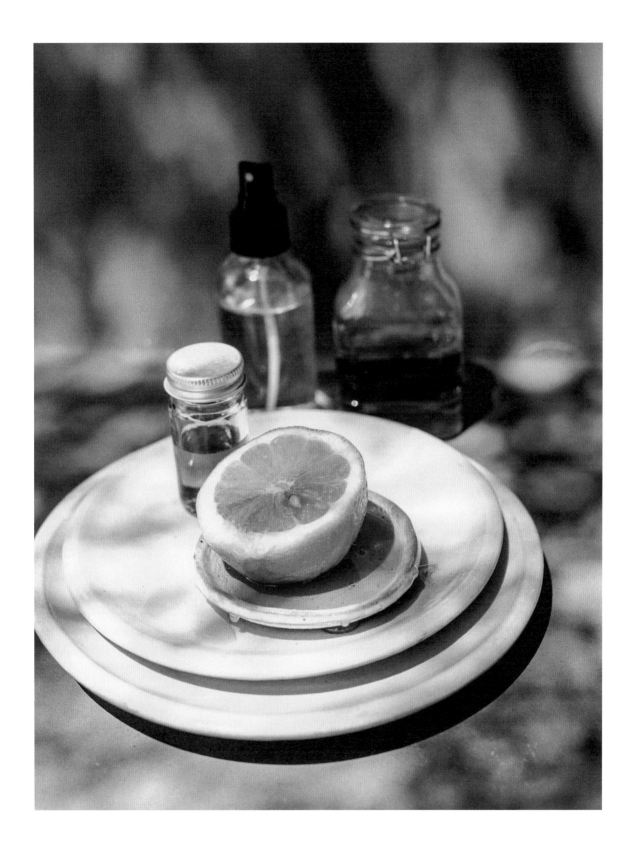

Nettle Leaf Nourishing Hair Tonic (Dry Hair)

A hydrating hair tonic that gives your scalp a deep clean.

TIME: 40 minutes

MAKES: 15.2 ounces (450 mL) hair tonic

YOU'LL NEED: a glass jar and a 16-ounce (480 mL) mist bottle

COMPONENTS

4 teaspoons loose nettle leaves or 2 nettle leaf tea bags

1¾ cups boiling filtered water

2 tablespoons apple cider vinegar

10 drops cedarwood essential oil

10 drops geranium essential oil

5 drops rosemary essential oil

This hair tonic is an easy, everyday hair rinse that helps nourish hair, especially in the winter months or in drier, colder climates. Nettles are a weed that grows in places we wouldn't normally want things to grow, but once they're picked, they're a hugely beneficial herb. Nettles have highly astringent leaves that make them great for the skin and hair. Pairing the benefits of the nettle leaf with the apple cider vinegar helps tone the hair and get the scalp clean and prepared for better hair growth. The essential oils used in this tonic are great for a calming, grounding energy and an aroma that is both fresh and earthy. I love using this tonic in the morning before or after my shampoo.

METHOD

1. In a glass jar, steep the nettle leaves or tea bags in boiling water for 15 to 20 minutes. Strain the leaves or remove the tea bag. Pour the tea into a mist bottle.
2. Allow the tea to cool completely, then add the apple cider vinegar (it's important to let the mixture cool first or else the vinegar will evaporate).
3. Add all essential oils.
4. Shake gently to combine.

APPLICATION

1. Shake gently before using.
2. Spray the tonic all over wet hair (or pour about ¼ cup over wet hair) before or after you apply shampoo (depending on preference).
3. Using your fingertips, massage the tonic into the scalp and comb it through your hair for best results.
4. Continue with shampoo and conditioner as desired.
5. For best results, use once a week.

STORAGE

Keep in a cool, dry place for up to 1 week or in the fridge for up to 2 weeks.

Lemongrass Lightening Hair Tonic (Oily Hair)

A tonic that naturally lightens your hair and gets you outdoors. Win-win.

TIME: 5 minutes + 30 to 90 minutes for processing
MAKES: 9.3 ounces (275 mL) hair tonic
YOU'LL NEED: a 12-ounce (360 mL) mist bottle

COMPONENTS

¼ cup freshly squeezed lemon juice

¾ cup filtered water

2 tablespoons organic liquid honey

3 drops lemongrass essential oil

3 drops peppermint essential oil

This hair tonic is perfect for the summer, especially for those who want to naturally lighten their hair colour a bit. The lemon juice helps naturally control oil production on the scalp and leaves hair looking a little bit brighter if applied before a day in the sun on a hike or at the beach (which I highly suggest). I've used this tonic during the summer on multiple occasions, once after doing a quick dip in the ocean and another after bathing in a lake while camping. The benefit of this hair tonic is that you will likely have most of its components with you while camping or exploring anyways (except for the mist bottle—you might need to find that). I hope this fresh tonic evokes the feeling of summer and brings a sense of lightness to your mood.

METHOD

1. Add all components into a mist bottle (you may need to use a funnel).
2. Shake well to combine to help the honey dissipate throughout the mixture.

APPLICATION

1. Shake gently before using.
2. Spray the tonic all over wet hair (or pour about ¼ cup over wet hair).
3. Leave the tonic in your hair for 30 to 90 minutes (this time can be spent indoors or outside to get the full lightening benefits).
4. To remove, rinse the tonic out of your hair with a natural homemade shampoo or water and allow the hair to air-dry.
5. For best results, use once a week or twice a month.

STORAGE

Keep in a cool, dry place for up to 4 days or in the fridge for up to 2 weeks.

Rosemary Strengthening Hair Tonic (Colour-Treated Hair)

An herbal, soothing tonic for repairing and replenishing your hair.

TIME: 40 minutes

MAKES: 16 ounces (480 mL) hair tonic

YOU'LL NEED: a glass jar and a 16-ounce (480 mL) mist bottle

COMPONENTS

5 tablespoons chamomile leaves or 2 organic chamomile tea bags

Boiling filtered water

1 to 2 sprigs fresh rosemary

1 teaspoon apple cider vinegar

10 drops rosemary essential oil

This tonic for colour-treated hair can be used by anyone who wants a little pick-me-up in their hair routine. It's full of hydrating and strengthening herbs and essential oils that help build strength in the hair and scalp. With subtle herbal tones from the rosemary and slightly sweet and calming properties from the chamomile, this is a beautiful weekly ritual to flush out any buildup and keep your hair routine simple, effective and natural.

METHOD

1. In a glass jar, steep the chamomile leaves or tea bags and fresh rosemary in boiling water for 15 to 20 minutes.
2. Strain the tea into a mist bottle.
3. Allow the chamomile and rosemary mixture to cool, then add the apple cider vinegar (it's important to let the mixture cool first or else the vinegar will evaporate).
4. Add the rosemary essential oil.
5. Shake gently to combine.

APPLICATION

1. Shake gently before using.
2. Spray the tonic all over wet hair (or pour about ¼ cup over wet hair) before or after you apply shampoo (depending on preference).
3. Using your fingertips, massage the tonic into the scalp and comb it through your hair for best results.
4. Continue with shampoo and conditioner as desired.
5. For best results, use once a week.

STORAGE

Keep in a cool, dry place for up to 1 week or in the fridge for up to 2 weeks.

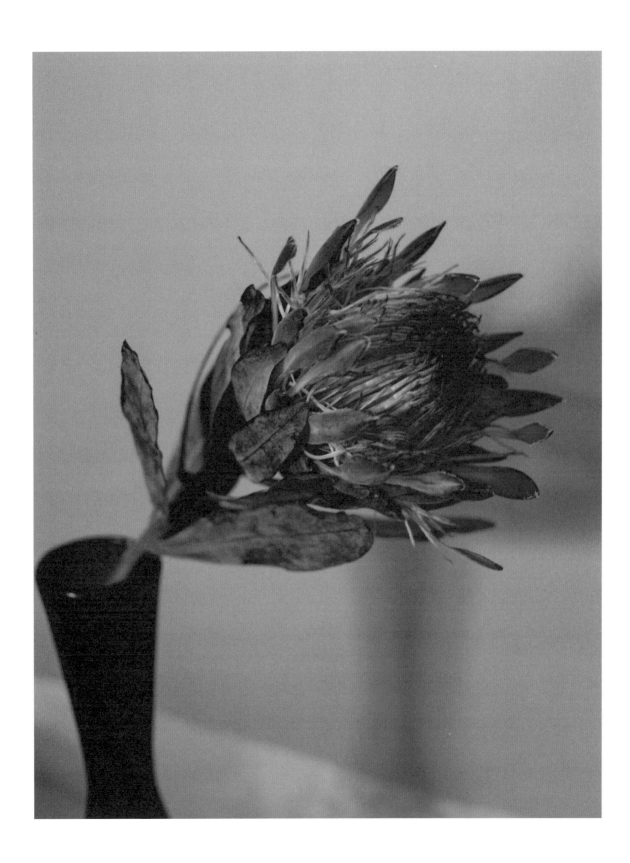

MORNING WHIPPED BODY BUTTERS

After a shower in the morning (especially after a workout), I want something to seal the fresh moisture into my skin, but I don't want a heavy body oil that could stain my clothing. In the morning, I opt for an easy to apply and even easier to make whipped body butter. These simple recipes allow for a light and fresh product, while still containing all the hydrating and moisturizing benefits of pure carrier oils. I love experimenting seasonally with different essential oils and usually switch between my Cloud 9 Ultra Whipped Body Butter (page 174) for the fall and winter months and my Easy Two-Ingredient Whipped Body Butter (page 175) during the spring and summer. I know that everyone says it, but your skin really is your largest organ, and the products and especially lotions you put on your body should nourish it in the best way with only the purest ingredients. This is such an easy switch to make in changing to natural products, and I hope you'll enjoy these dessert-like products as much as I do. They really do look like a beautiful whipped cream dessert. These recipes are also my favourites because my mom actually introduced me to whipped body butters; she's really awesome, and so are these.

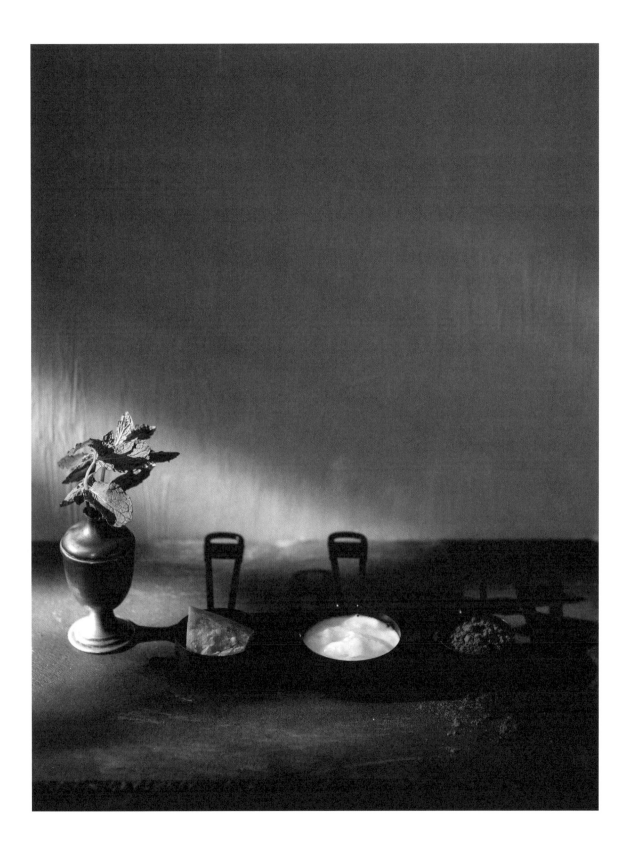

Cloud 9 Ultra Whipped Body Butter

Start your morning with dessert.

TIME: 45 minutes

MAKES: 8 ounces (240 mL) whipped body butter

YOU'LL NEED: a double boiler, a stand mixer and an 8-ounce (240 mL) container with a lid

COMPONENTS

¾ cup organic solid virgin coconut oil

¼ cup organic cocoa butter

1 teaspoon organic cocoa powder

10 drops peppermint essential oil

STORAGE

Keep in a cool, dark place away from direct sunlight for up to 2 months. If you live in a humid climate, keep in the fridge.

Who would have thought that you could slather yourself in a rich dessert-like cream before 9 am? I do this every morning (especially in the fall and winter months) with this mint chocolate whipped body butter. Body oils are my favourite way to hydrate my skin, but during the morning rush they can be messy and too time consuming, which is why I often just skip them all together. As a way of fixing this, I created this recipe that uses air to whip my favourite carrier oils and essential oils into a solid state that melts easily into the skin when applied to the body. The Cloud 9 recipe uses coconut oil as well as cocoa butter, which is even more hydrating and helps lock in more moisture than just plain coconut oil. During fall and winter months, I add cocoa powder and a couple of drops of peppermint because who doesn't want to be covered in a little chocolate mint aroma before getting dressed and taking on the day? It's a little secret indulgence I always appreciate before putting on my blazer and taking on the world.

METHOD

1. Using a double boiler, melt the coconut oil and cocoa butter until fully combined in a liquid state.
2. Remove from the heat and allow to cool for about 30 to 45 minutes (the liquid will become cloudy and the mixture should be cool to touch—if it takes too long, put it in the freezer for 30 minutes to speed up the process).
3. Once the combination has solidified and is cool to the touch, in the bowl of a stand mixer with the whisk attachment or an electric mixer (which will take a little more arm muscle), whip the solid butter mixture on maximum speed for 3 minutes or until the mixture starts to form solid peaks.
4. When the body butter starts to change consistency, add the cocoa powder and peppermint essential oil.
5. Continue mixing for 2 to 3 minutes or until the body butter and cocoa powder are well combined and achieve the consistency of whipped cream or fluffy white clouds.
6. Gently spoon the whipped body butter into a container with a lid.

APPLICATION

1. Using your fingers or a spoon, scoop out the whipped body butter 1 tablespoon at a time and spread a thin layer evenly over your body. The body butter will melt when it touches your skin.
2. Let dry for a few minutes to ensure that your clothing doesn't get stained. I love applying the body butter after the shower and then wrapping myself in a towel to do my hair and makeup before getting dressed.

Easy Two-Ingredient Whipped Body Butter

A "choose your own adventure" body butter experience.

TIME: 10 minutes

MAKES: 8 ounces (240 mL) whipped body butter

YOU'LL NEED: a stand mixer and an 8-ounce (240 mL) container with lid

COMPONENTS

1 cup organic solid virgin coconut oil

10 drops of your favourite essential oil

The perfect summer body moisturizer, this light-as-air whipped body butter has only two ingredients: coconut oil and whatever essential oil you want to add. I love using fresher aromas for this body butter because the sweet summer aroma of coconut really comes through with the simplicity of this formula. For product ideas, try mixing a few drops of lemongrass essential oil or geranium essential oil for a more goddess-like aroma. Or, if you want to keep things really simple, make this a one-ingredient body butter by leaving out the essential oil. This body butter is super easy to make and to switch up by creating your own custom aroma that sinks right into the skin.

METHOD

1. In the bowl of a stand mixer with the whisk attachment, add the coconut oil and essential oil and whip on maximum speed for 6 to 7 minutes or until the mixture starts to form solid peaks like whipping cream.
2. Gently scoop the whipped body butter into a container with a lid.

APPLICATION

1. Using your fingers or a spoon, scoop out the whipped body butter 1 tablespoon at a time and spread a thin layer evenly over your body. The body butter will melt when it touches your skin.
2. Let dry for a few minutes to ensure that your clothing doesn't get stained. I love applying the body butter after the shower and then wrapping myself in a towel to do my hair and makeup before getting dressed.

STORAGE

Keep in a cool, dark place away from direct sunlight for up to 2 months. If you live in a humid climate, keep in the fridge.

FOR THE BOYS

Essential oils are products that are versatile enough for anyone. Their aromas and benefits make them easy to use in the medicine cabinets and makeup or shaving kits of men and women alike. The following recipes are an easy introduction to the world of essential oils for men. Simple and cost effective, these recipes can help men replace some of the more traditional products in their bathrooms with natural alternatives that work just as effectively.

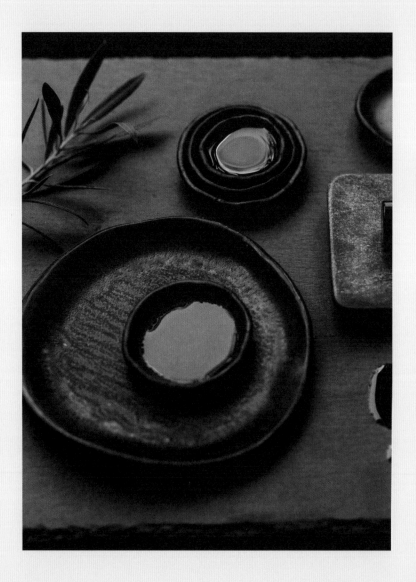

Aftershave

A gentle treatment that soothes sensitive, freshly shaved skin.

TIME: 3 minutes

MAKES: 2.87 ounces (85 mL) aftershave

YOU'LL NEED: a 3-ounce (90 mL) mist bottle

COMPONENTS

2 tablespoons non-alcoholic witch hazel

2 tablespoons organic aloe vera gel

1 tablespoon filtered water

2 teaspoons pomegranate seed oil

2 to 3 drops lavender essential oil

2 to 3 drops rosemary essential oil

2 drops cedarwood essential oil

1 drop frankincense essential oil

Many men experience irritation from the synthetic fragrances and strong alcohols used in traditional aftershaves. Switching to a natural aftershave that has gentle yet effective plant-derived ingredients can have the same results as traditional aftershave, without the potential of irritated skin.

METHOD

1. In a mist bottle, add the witch hazel, aloe vera gel and water and shake well to combine.
2. Add the pomegranate seed oil and all essential oils.

APPLICATION

1. Shake well before each use to ensure that the components are evenly distributed.
2. After shaving, close the eyes and mist the face. Gently pat the mixture into the face, focusing on the cheeks, chin and neck.

STORAGE

Keep in a cool, dry place for up to 1 month.

Beard Oil

A moisturizing treatment to keep your beard happy and healthy.

TIME: 5 minutes

MAKES: 2.5 ounces (75 mL) oil

YOU'LL NEED: a 3-ounce (90 mL) dropper bottle

COMPONENTS

3 tablespoons jojoba oil

2 tablespoons sweet almond oil

10 drops cedarwood essential oil

4 drops rosemary essential oil

2 drops geranium essential oil

2 drops frankincense essential oil

Beard oils have become popular in recent years since the beard itself has made a comeback. Buying beard oil at a trendy store can be quite expensive, so making your own at home is a great alternative and allows the scent to be completely customized for you.

METHOD

1. Add all components to a dropper bottle.
2. Place the cap on tightly and shake gently to combine.

APPLICATION

1. To use, apply 2 to 5 drops of beard oil (depending on the texture and density of the hair) to your hands and then massage into the beard and the face, if desired.

STORAGE

Keep in a cool, dry place for up to 1 month.

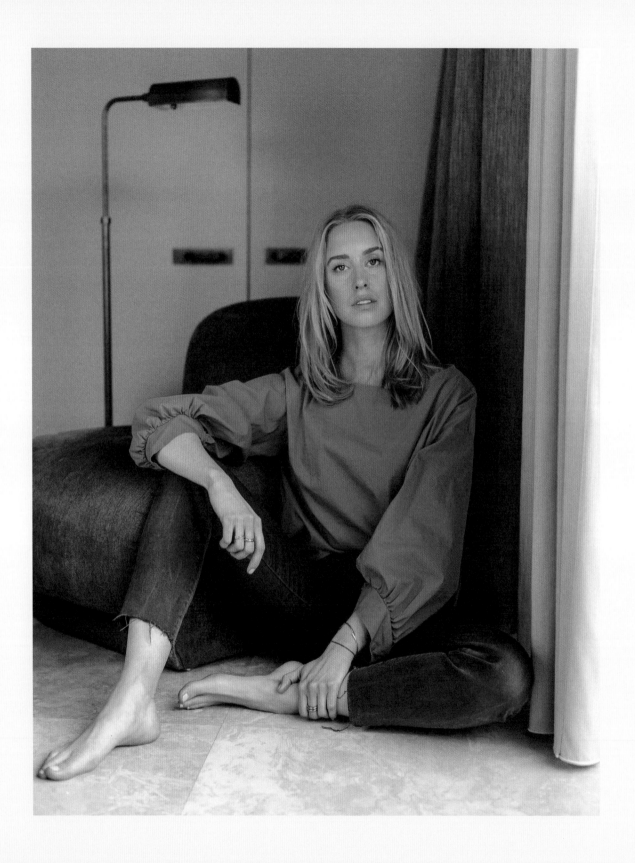

AFTERNOON BODY RITUALS

The afternoon is when I tend to dissociate from my body and its needs. After a couple of hours at my desk, looking at a computer or running between meetings and living mostly in my head, I find that the afternoon is the most important time for practices that remind me to breathe. It's these moments when I need to feel grounded and get back to centre. In this section, I've shared some of the easy ways I use products and habits throughout my afternoon as a means of cueing my brain and body to get back into alignment and in the zone. Most of these have been created out of necessity, wanting to ensure I am focused, energized and present for our team (or whomever I'm spending the afternoon with).

I invite you to experiment with some of these habits and slot them into different moments of your afternoon (especially around the 3 pm slump). It's pretty incredible what we can do for our brains and bodies by having a little extra water in our system and some natural essential oils to cue our alertness.

Body Mists

TIME: 2 minutes

MAKES: 2 ounces (60 mL) body mist

YOU'LL NEED: a 2-ounce (60 mL) mist bottle

COMPONENTS

2 tablespoons filtered water

3 teaspoons witch hazel

3 teaspoons pomegranate seed oil (optional)

Your favourite body mist blend (see page 182)

I'm not sure about you, but most of my day is spent on my feet going from meeting to meeting, running after my dog or squeezing in a jog after a long workday before dashing to a late dinner reservation. My purpose in sharing this is that some days are easier than others to fit in a second shower; on many days I don't have time to go home and wash off before an evening date or business dinner. It's during these busy moments that I love incorporating homemade body mists. I jokingly call them a "shower in a bottle," but they truly are.

This is a simple formulation to help you freshen up as you go. Below is the standard formulation for the body mist, which you can then customize seasonally or switch up based on your climate.

METHOD
1. Add all components to a mist bottle.
2. Shake well.

APPLICATION
1. Shake well before each use.
2. Mist over your body (over and/or under your shirt), neck and back throughout the day as desired. This product is also safe to mist over the face if the eyes are closed.
3. Breathe deeply, and stretch a bit if you have time (or at least stretch your arms).

STORAGE
Keep in a mist bottle away from direct sunlight and extreme temperature changes for up to 1 month. For an extra-refreshing mist, keep in the refrigerator.

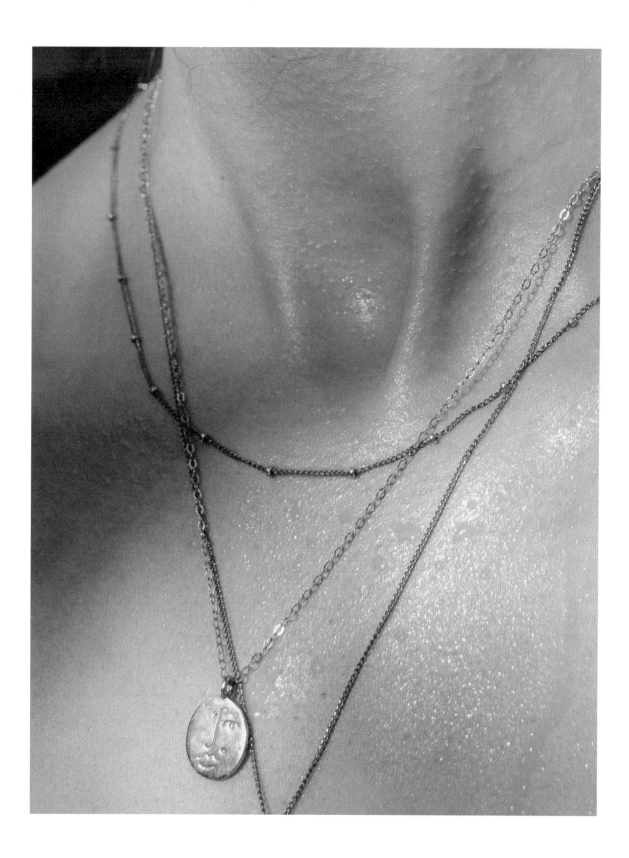

Essential Oil Aroma Blends for Body Mists

BOSS BODY MIST
For when you need to be (or at least smell) in charge.
10 drops cedarwood essential oil
5 drops geranium essential oil
5 drops rosemary essential oil

Keep at your desk.

AFTER THE RAIN BODY MIST
A modern take on a traditional deodorant aroma.
10 drops spruce essential oil
5 drops ylang ylang essential oil
5 drops tea tree essential oil

Keep in your car.

OH, HEY YOU BODY MIST
For when you're around people you really like.
10 drops cedarwood essential oil
5 drops bergamot essential oil
3 drops frankincense essential oil
2 drops grapefruit essential oil

Keep in your purse (you never know where you might end up or who you might run in to).

SPA SHOWER IN A BOTTLE BODY MIST
For when your next spa visit is nowhere in sight.
10 drops eucalyptus essential oil
5 drops peppermint essential oil
5 drops lemon essential oil

Keep in your bathroom or office bathroom—wherever you need to start smelling like you just walked out of an invigorating spa treatment.

On-the-Go Cuticle and Hand Oils

TIME: 2 minutes

MAKES: 0.17 ounce (5 mL) cuticle oil

YOU'LL NEED: a 0.3-ounce (10 mL) dropper bottle

COMPONENTS

Your favourite cuticle and hand oil blend (see page 184)

The secret to healthy-looking hands and manicures that last longer? Cuticle oil. I've recently become a huge fan of cuticle oil and now have a few different dropper bottles in my car, in my purse and beside my bed, so that I can keep up my habit of hydrating and nourishing my nails while I'm on the go.

If you really want to maintain that glow you get after a professional manicure, cuticle oil is your answer. Sure, the perfectly applied polish seems like the star of the show, but the real secret is often the cuticle and nail oil they use at the end of the appointment. Moisturizing your cuticles and doing a simple reflexology massage on your hands is an easy way to de-stress and keep the hands looking healthy and nourished while you're on the move.

METHOD

1. Add all components to a dropper bottle.

APPLICATION

1. Apply 1 drop of oil to the base of each nail bed on one hand (or ½ drop if nails and cuticles are not very dry).
2. Using the other hand, massage the oil into each nail, applying gentle pressure to the nail bed as you massage.
3. Repeat on the other hand.

STORAGE

Keep in a cool, dry place away from direct sunlight (or in your bag when you're out and about) for up to 1 month.

Essential Oil Aroma Blends for Cuticle and Hand Oils

WINTER WOODS CUTICLE AND HAND OIL

A cozy aroma with depth that warms you up.

1 teaspoon sweet almond oil

5 drops cedarwood essential oil

3 drops bergamot essential oil

SPRING FLORAL CUTICLE AND HAND OIL

A delicate and floral aroma that channels your feminine energy.

1 teaspoon apricot seed oil

5 drops geranium essential oil

3 drops ylang ylang essential oil

SUMMER CITRUS CUTICLE AND HAND OIL

A bright, citrusy aroma (to match that coral nail colour you chose).

1 teaspoon grapeseed oil

5 drops grapefruit essential oil

3 drops lemon essential oil

FALL HERBAL CUTICLE AND HAND OIL

A fresh and herbal aroma that's like a reawakening for your hands.

1 teaspoon jojoba oil

5 drops peppermint essential oil

3 drops lavender essential oil

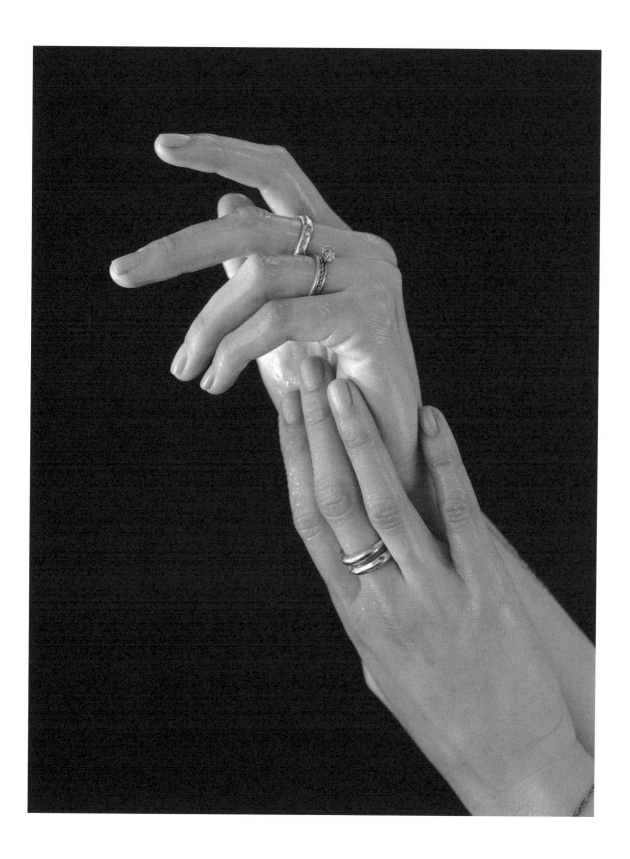

Salves for Everything

TIME: 10 minutes

MAKES: 2.5 ounces (75 mL) salve

YOU'LL NEED: a double boiler, a metal or wooden spoon and a 3-ounce (90 mL) container with a lid

COMPONENTS

2 tablespoons organic shea butter

2 tablespoons beeswax, grated or in pellets (it won't melt at the right speed if it's a solid chunk)

1 tablespoon sweet almond oil or jojoba oil

Your favourite salve blend (see page 187)

Salves are a great way to incorporate essential oils into the everyday hustle in a way that's slightly more portable and travel friendly. They are created by taking a solid (like beeswax) and a liquid (like sweet almond oil or jojoba oil) and combining them in ratios that result in a semi-solid formulation that stays solid on its own but melts into the skin when applied. They take slightly longer to make in comparison to some of the other formulations in this book, but the great thing about them is that they are super concentrated and last for a really long time. With salves, a little goes a very long way.

METHOD

1. In a double boiler, add the shea butter, beeswax and sweet almond or jojoba oil and stir with a metal or wooden spoon until it just melts (ensure that it doesn't overheat).
2. As soon as the mixture is fully combined, remove from heat.
3. Allow to cool for 1 to 3 minutes, then pour into the container (leaving the lid off).
4. Once the mixture has slightly cooled (the colour will change from clear to opaque), add the salve blend. Allowing the mixture to cool slightly first ensures that the volatile oils in the essential oils will not evaporate from the heat.
5. Allow the container to cool overnight (letting all the moisture evaporate), then store with the lid on and carry it around as needed.

APPLICATION

1. Using a spoon or your fingers, take less than 1 teaspoon of the salve at a time and rub into the skin where desired.

STORAGE

Keep in a cool, dark place for up to 3 months. If you live in a warm climate, keeping it in the fridge is best.

Essential Oil Aroma Blends for Salves

NECK AND SHOULDER SALVE

For computer shoulders.

10 drops eucalyptus essential oil

10 drops peppermint essential oil

3 drops spruce essential oil

2 drops tea tree essential oil

Keep at your desk.

HAND SALVE

For saving the world.

10 drops frankincense essential oil

5 drops geranium essential oil

5 drops grapefruit essential oil

Keep in your bag.

CUTICLE AND BROW SALVE

For all the things.

10 drops rosemary essential oil

5 drops ylang ylang essential oil

5 drops frankincense essential oil

Keep with your toiletries and makeup.

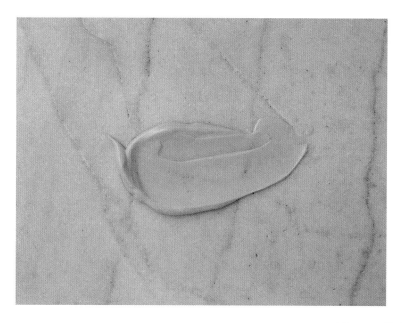

WEEKEND POWER NAP

I've recently become a fan of the weekend power nap. I've started taking them on Saturdays, Sundays or long weekends when there's the luxury of time and the sun is hitting the living room just right at 3 pm. I close my eyes for 20 minutes of blissfully deep sleep—it's just enough time to help you recharge but not so much that you feel groggy afterwards. Cultures all around the world specifically create times in each day for people to naturally have a quick nap or siesta. Here are a few of my favourite ways to set the mood and create the perfect state for napping and the modern siesta.

1. COVER YOUR EYES

When napping in the middle of the day (or late afternoon), I love using a silk eye cover that keeps any eye makeup I have in place and helps to naturally shut out any sunlight. The silk fabric usually stays cooler, which also helps relieve puffiness around the eyes.

2. SCENT

Pairing a nap with an aroma that helps promote deep breathing is my favourite way to cue the brain and body that it's time for a quick snooze. I love using organic eucalyptus oil because not only does it smell like a spa, but it also prompts me to take full, deep breaths. I also love using it for naps, because it's relaxing but not in a sedative way. To use scent while napping, I set up a diffuser beside the couch or wherever I'm taking my nap. If I'm travelling or on the go, I simply add 1 to 2 drops of eucalyptus essential oil to the nose area of my eye mask or add 1 drop topically under my nose.

3. HEAVY BLANKET

It may seem excessive, but having a nice, heavy blanket can help quiet the brain's chatter and remind the body to slow down and rest. I love using a heavy linen blanket or, in the summer months, a light Turkish towel-style blanket that creates a sense of coziness without being overly warm.

4. PEPPERMINT TEA

Hydration is key before and after a nap. I love making a pot or just a cup of peppermint tea and drinking half before my nap and finishing it after I wake up. Hydrating the body and mind before and after a nap helps increase the natural cognitive benefits of the nap, and it's also important to rehydrate after you've been sleeping.

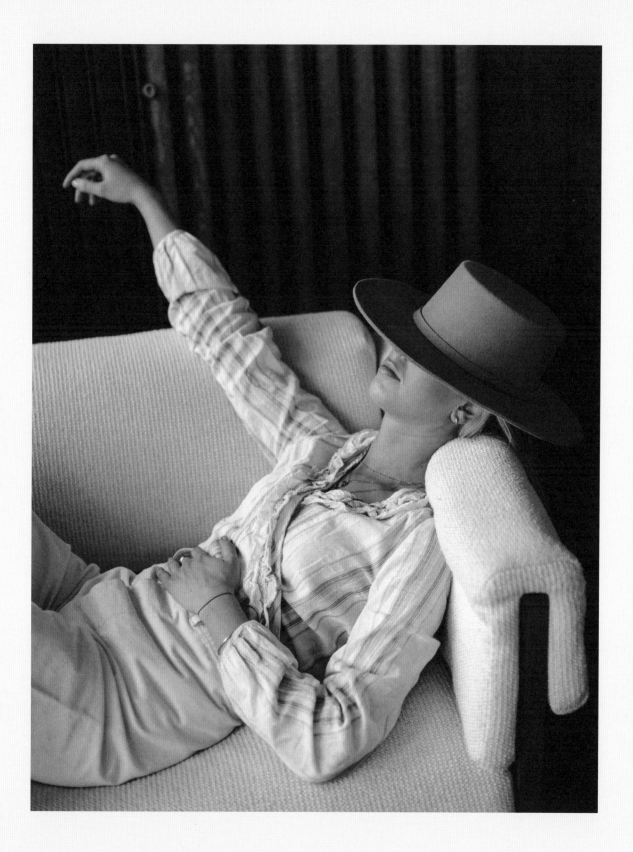

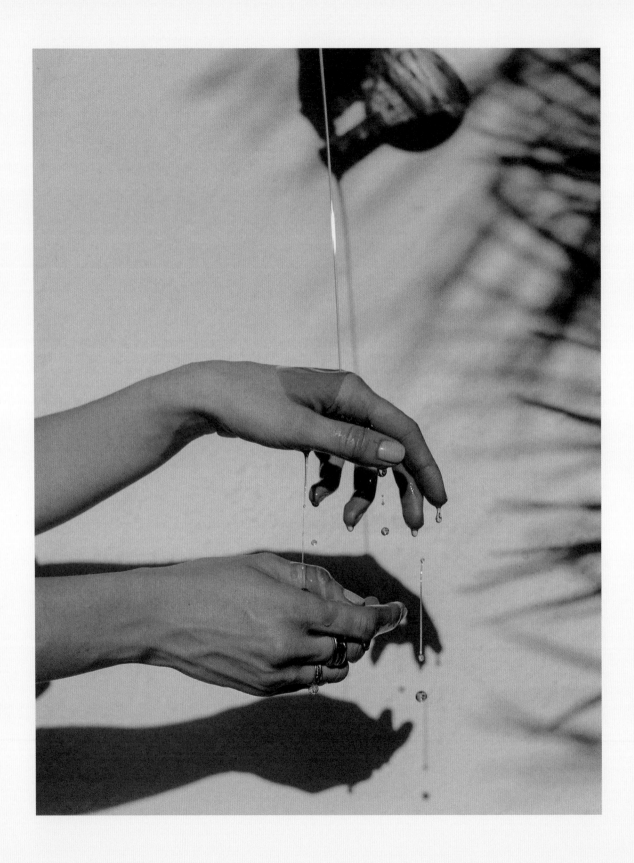

EVENING BODY RITUALS

The evening is possibly the easiest time to establish rituals. For me, these rituals have become reminders to return to an awareness of my body after living in my head for most of the day. Creating simple and discrete ways to reconnect with my body has helped slow my busy brain before going to sleep. Awareness of the body doesn't mean analysis or judgment but the very opposite: gratitude and appreciation. Gratitude for the vessel that got me through the day, walked me to meetings, ran after my dog—the thing that gives me life and breath to be present and alert. This may sound a little heavy, but it really is something I have worked on over the years. When you have work that you love, passion and vision, the body becomes something you want to nurture and look after, so that you can experience your goals and your vision. The body isn't the destination, it's the means by which we flow through life. And for that reason, I find as much time as I can in the simple moments of my day to take care of it, so that I can do the work I do in the ways that I do it—fast, intense and relentless. To counteract that drive, some foot soaks, hair masks and bath oils are necessary. I hope these simple recipes give you and your body a little more fuel to get back out there and create what you envision.

LATE NIGHT HAIR MASKS

During the week, I keep my beauty and body routine very simple; I wake up, rinse my face and apply a light oil moisturizer. In the evenings, I keep my routine to less than three products, but Sunday is when I do the most in preparation for the week ahead. I've been this way for years, and it's become a sacred time for recharging. My Sunday night rituals make me feel mentally and physically refreshed and ready for whatever Monday morning will bring.

For me, the perfect Sunday night is spent with a hydrating hair mask. It's a simple indulgence that usually happens while I'm planning the week ahead or clearing out an inbox late on a Sunday. I'd even say it's best enjoyed accompanied by a bath and a glass of wine. Here are two of my favourite hair masks, along with notes on when I use them. Nourishing the hair is something that women have done for centuries. In Ayurvedic practices, they would use warm oil associated with your dosha. Clay masks for the hair are used throughout sub-Saharan Africa, and shea butter is applied to the skin and hair in cultures around the world. The act of nourishing ourselves by applying masks is one of the oldest traditions in beauty. I hope these modern versions of ancient rituals bring some gentle and grounding energy to your evening routine.

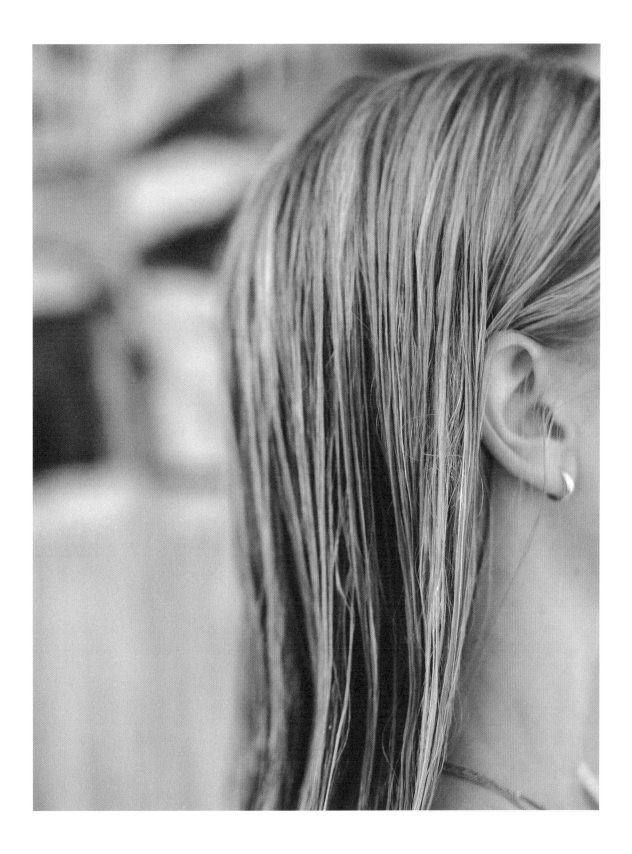

Sunday Night Hair Mask

A hydrating hair mask to finish off the week.

TIME: 2 minutes to make; leave on for 30 to 60 minutes
MAKES: 1 hair mask
YOU'LL NEED: a small bowl

COMPONENTS

2 teaspoons sweet almond oil

2 teaspoons avocado oil

2 teaspoons organic solid virgin coconut oil

10 drops rosemary essential oil

5 drops cedarwood essential oil

2 drops peppermint essential oil

The most conditioning hair mask I've ever used, this simple recipe is best left on for 30 minutes to 1 hour and somehow always seems to work better when paired with a great movie and a cup of tea (or a glass of wine) on a Sunday night. Regardless of the relaxation you build around it, this mask has become a staple in my weekly routine, and I try to do it at least twice a month to give my hair some needed TLC. I especially love this mask when I've been adding more heat damage to my hair with a curling iron. The quantities in this recipe work for short to medium-length hair—if your hair is longer or quite thick, try doubling the recipe. Dare I say it, pair this hair mask with your favourite face mask . . .

METHOD

1. Mix together all components in a small bowl.

APPLICATION

1. On dry or wet hair, apply 1 teaspoon at a time, starting at the roots and massaging into the scalp.
2. Comb throughout the hair, ensuring you get the oil to the ends of your hair.
3. If possible, braid or swirl your hair into a loose bun and tie it back to make sure the oil doesn't get on your clothing or furniture. If your hair is too short for this, it's fine to leave it down.
4. Leave the mask in hair for 30 to 60 minutes, then rinse out with shampoo in the shower if you have more fine hair. If you have thicker, coarser hair, you can leave the mask on without rinsing it out.

STORAGE

If making larger quantities of the hair mask, keep in a container with a lid in a cool, dry place for up to 2 months.

Secret Moisturizing Hair Mask

A super-nourishing hair mask you can wear on the go.

TIME: 2 minutes to make

MAKES: 1 hair mask

YOU'LL NEED: a small bowl

COMPONENTS

1 teaspoon grapeseed oil

1 teaspoon apricot kernel oil

10 drops rosemary essential oil

5 drops cedarwood essential oil

2 drops geranium essential oil

This is a lighter version of a hair mask that's great for dry or damaged hair. It's a formula I bring with me in a small dropper bottle and apply to the ends of my hair while travelling. It's helpful when you're on a plane or even for daily use if your hair is feeling extra dry. All you have to do is apply it to the ends and swirl your hair into a low bun. No one will know you're secretly strengthening and hydrating your hair, and you'll look very Parisian chic. Feel free to experiment with the aromas of this oil, but rosemary essential oil should always be the base because of its positive and strengthening effects on the hair. The quantities in this recipe work for short to medium-length hair—if your hair is longer or quite thick, try doubling the recipe.

METHOD

1. Mix together all components in a small bowl.

APPLICATION

1. On dry hair, apply to ends of the hair and comb it through.
2. If possible, braid or swirl your hair into a loose bun and tie it back to make sure the oil doesn't get on your clothing or furniture. If your hair is too short for this, it's fine to leave it down.

STORAGE

If making larger quantities of the hair mask, keep in a dropper bottle in a cool, dry place for up to 2 months.

FOOT SOAKS FOR TIRED FEET

I once received three missed calls from my mom in a row and felt a wave of anxiety that something was wrong. I immediately called her back, only to hear water splashing on the other end of the phone and her saying, "Hon, I just created the most amazing foot soak for after work!" I was slightly less enthusiastic than I think she wanted me to be but was very relieved she was calling about a relaxing foot soak and not a family emergency.

Since that call, foot soaks have become part of my evening ritual after work. My mom introduced me to them when I was growing up—she is an elementary school teacher and would be on her feet all day long with the kids. Upon coming home, she would take 5 minutes to draw herself a bit of warm water in the bath and soak her feet. She also taught me the importance of blood flow and making time to elevate your feet when you can, especially when you're on them all day. I'm not a schoolteacher, but I have the pleasure of working at a bustling and very dynamic office where I am usually up and out of my chair a few times an hour. If there's any evening ritual I would suggest implementing right away, it's the simple pleasure of soaking your feet after work. It doesn't need to be completely luxurious—I often end up simply sitting on the side of the bathtub with my pants rolled up answering emails on my phone. But if you can carve out even just a few more minutes, it can be a lovely way to get the body and brain to *let go* and soak away all that you carried with you during the day. Patting your feet dry after a foot soak is a fresh start, and the evening is yours.

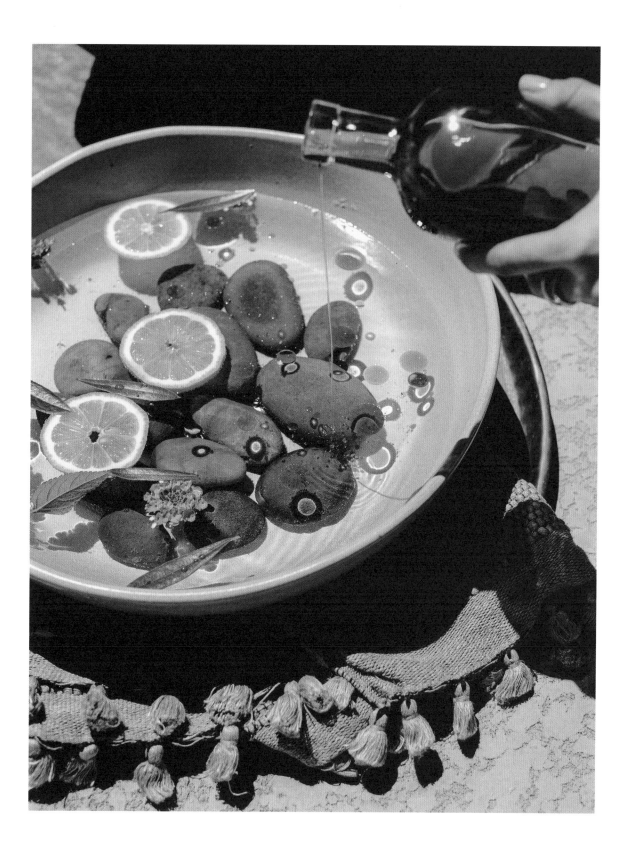

Rejuvenating Ginger and Peppermint Foot Soak

A refreshing foot soak that brings life back to tired feet.

TIME: 10 minutes

MAKES: 1 foot soak

YOU'LL NEED: a water basin (optional), a small towel and 10 smooth rocks (optional)

COMPONENTS

1-inch piece peeled fresh ginger

7 drops peppermint essential oil

Warming and cooling for any time of the year, the combination of botanicals and roots make this a natural hot and cold treatment for the feet. The fresh ginger is warming and can help improve blood circulation to the feet while also detoxifying. The peppermint essential oil has naturally cooling properties and has also been shown to have antibacterial and anti-inflammatory properties—particularly useful during the summer months for tired, swollen feet that may have been sweating.

METHOD

1. Grate or finely chop the ginger. Reserve as much of the ginger liquid as possible.
2. Fill a bathtub with 2 to 3 inches of warm water or until your feet are fully submerged. If you don't want to use a bathtub, use a water basin filled with warm water and a comfortable chair to sit in.
3. Add the ginger, any reserved ginger liquid and peppermint essential oil to the warm water.

APPLICATION

1. Soak your feet in the warm water.
2. If using a basin, try adding 5 to 10 smooth rocks that you can use to massage your feet.
3. Keep your feet submerged for as long as you need.
4. Breathe deeply, try some calf stretches and take a few moments for yourself.

Lemon and Olive Spanish Foot Soak

A rich and hydrating Mediterranean-inspired foot soak.

TIME: 10 minutes

MAKES: 1 foot soak

YOU'LL NEED: a water basin (optional), a small towel and 10 smooth rocks (optional)

COMPONENTS

10 drops lemon essential oil

2 teaspoons olive oil

1 teaspoon salt

This foot soak was inspired by the time I spent in Spain, eating far too many olives and enjoying them with the freshness of lemon. I created this soak one day in a hotel bathroom after a flight from Portugal. I needed my feet to feel a little more fresh before a day of walking, so I sat on the hotel bathroom counter, added a few drops of lemon essential oil and olive oil to the sink and soaked my feet. Simple, fresh and great for all seasons, this Spanish foot bath brings a little bit of the Mediterranean to wherever you are.

METHOD

1. Fill a bathtub with 2 to 3 inches of warm water or until your feet are fully submerged. If you don't want to use a bathtub, use a water basin filled with warm water and a comfortable chair to sit in.
2. Add the lemon essential oil, olive oil and salt to the warm water.

APPLICATION

1. Soak your feet in the warm water.
2. If using a basin, try adding 5 to 10 smooth rocks that you can use to massage your feet.
3. Keep your feet submerged for as long as you need.
4. Breathe deeply, try some calf stretches and take a few moments for yourself.
5. When you've finished, make sure to wipe the bathtub clean, as the olive oil will have left it slippery.

Whipped Body Creams

TIME: 10 minutes

MAKES: 8.45 ounces (250 mL) whipped body butter

YOU'LL NEED: a stand mixer and a dark glass or metal jar with a lid

COMPONENTS

1 cup organic solid virgin coconut oil

Your favourite essential oil aroma blend (see page 202)

All-natural ingredients can be formulated in ways that make them unexpected and a little more plush. Whipped body creams provide a lightweight texture but a deeply hydrating effect because they take rich, natural moisturizers and put air into them—much like how whipping cream is made in baking. The evening is an especially nice time to use whipped body creams because they need the natural heat from the body to melt into the skin. This makes them feel extra luxurious after a warm evening bath. Here is the simple formula for making them, followed by a few custom essential oil blends that work to balance the sweetness of the coconut oil.

METHOD

1. In the bowl of a stand mixer with the whisk attachment, whisk the coconut oil and essential oils on the highest speed until the mixture starts to form solid peaks like whipping cream, about 6 to 7 minutes.
2. Gently scoop the whipped body cream into a glass or metal jar with a lid.

APPLICATION

1. Using your fingers or a spoon, scoop out the whipped body cream 1 tablespoon at a time and spread a thin layer evenly over your body. The body cream will melt when it touches your skin.
2. Let dry for a few minutes to ensure that your clothing doesn't get stained. I love applying the body cream after an evening bath and then wrapping myself in a towel while I get ready for bed. This allows the full benefit of the moisture to sink in.

STORAGE

Keep in a cool, dark place away from direct sunlight for up to 2 months. If you live in a humid climate, store it in the fridge.

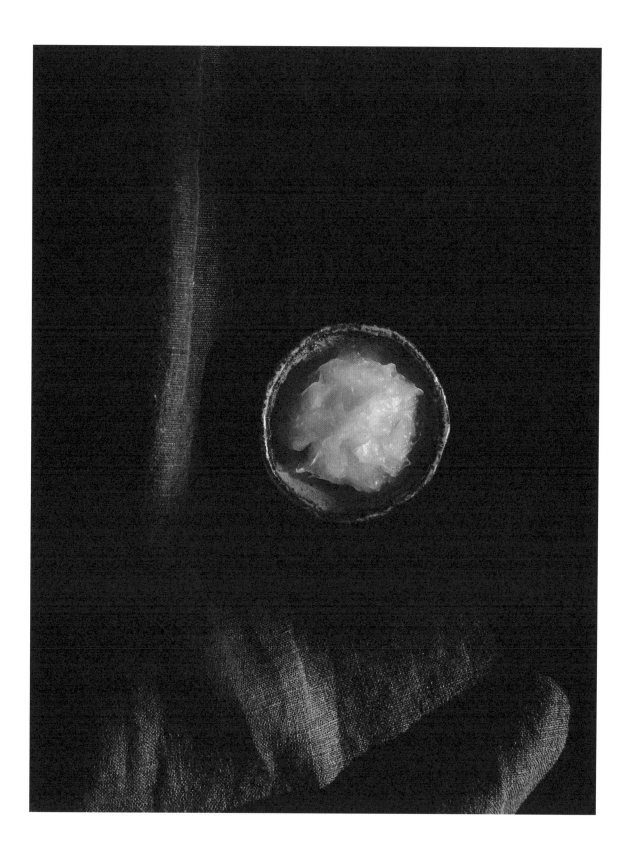

Essential Oil Aroma Blends for Whipped Body Creams

SMOKY AND SWEET

A dynamic aroma that's incredibly cozy yet fresh.

6 drops cedarwood essential oil

2 drops geranium essential oil

2 drops frankincense essential oil

WEST COAST ROOTS

The perfect way to ground your body before bed.

5 drops spruce essential oil

3 drops frankincense essential oil

2 drops lemon essential oil

THE LAND OF LAVENDER AND HONEY

Super indulgent and rich—just what your body needs.

1 teaspoon organic liquid honey

10 drops lavender essential oil

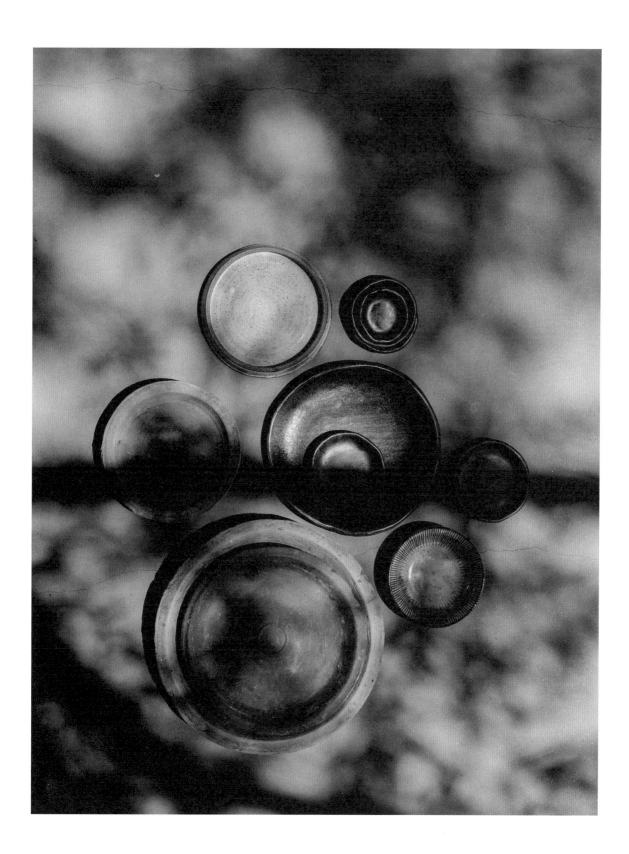

COMPLETELY CALMING TEA

Creating a healthy and restful sleep starts hours before you get into bed. The brain and body crave consistency and are always looking for cues and reminders of habits they find familiar. The ritual of sipping warm tea, its aroma and the calming effects of the dried botanicals all contribute to a habit that the brain and body can associate with sleep, which cues them to be aware of this shift in the day. This tea is a combination of some of my favourite herbs for creating a bit of calm at the end of the day, regardless of what has been thrown at you. Fennel, peppermint and ginger all aid in promoting healthy and calm digestion, which is a key component for getting a restful sleep. Lemon balm and lavender are very calming, and their aroma helps soothe and restore. You should be able to find all the ingredients used in this recipe at a grocery store. Whenever possible, try to choose organic ingredients.

TIME: 15 minutes

MAKES: 2 cups of tea

YOU'LL NEED: a small pot

INGREDIENTS

2 to 3 cups filtered water

1 tablespoon dried or fresh lemon balm

2 teaspoons dried or fresh peppermint leaves

1 teaspoon fennel seeds

1 teaspoon dried lavender flowers

2 slices peeled fresh ginger

2 teaspoons organic liquid honey, more as desired

Unsweetened almond milk, cashew milk or your favourite non-dairy milk

METHOD

1. In a small pot, bring the water to a boil, then add the lemon balm, peppermint, fennel, lavender and ginger and boil for 5 minutes.
2. Remove the pot from the stove and let the mixture steep for 2 to 4 minutes.
3. Strain the tea and discard the herbs.
4. Pour into cups and add honey and almond milk as desired.

STORAGE

This recipe makes enough for 2 cups of tea, so you can drink 1 cup and then store the other cup in the fridge for up to 4 days, to be reheated later or enjoyed iced on a hot summer night.

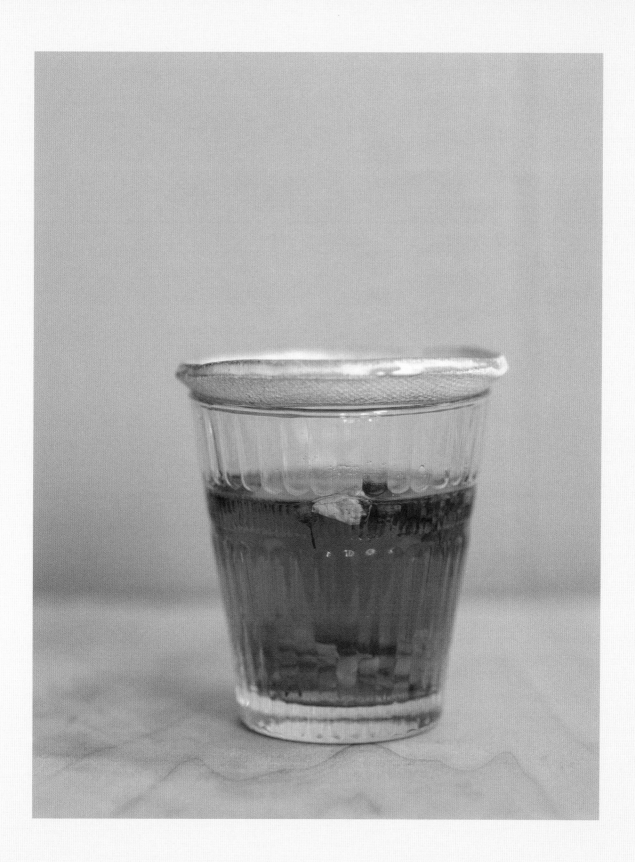

EVENING BODY SCRUBS

There's a significant difference between a body scrub for the morning and one for the evening—not only in the aroma chosen (to either relax or uplift), but also in the carrier oils and moisture levels. These evening body scrubs are formulated with a more deeply exfoliating sugar mixture, which provides a deeper clean and is paired with a more nourishing carrier oil to replenish and lock in moisture during your sleep cycle.

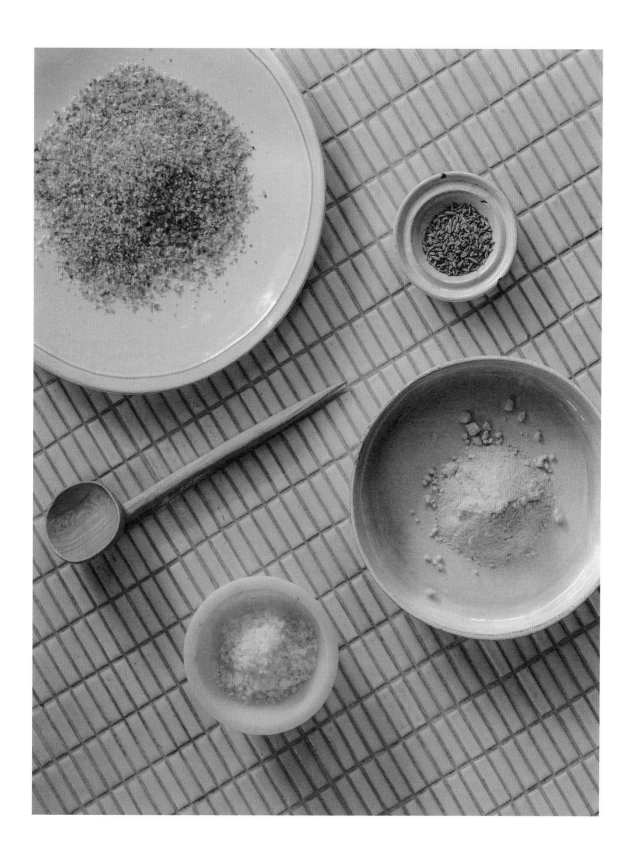

Warming Evening Body Scrub

A cozy scrub that leaves you smelling delicious.

TIME: 10 minutes

MAKES: 8 ounces (240 mL) scrub

YOU'LL NEED: a small bowl and an 8-ounce (240 mL) container with a lid

COMPONENTS

½ cup sugar

1 teaspoon cinnamon

½ cup apricot kernel oil

10 drops frankincense essential oil

10 drops cedarwood essential oil

5 drops bergamot essential oil

It doesn't get more cozy than this warming body scrub. Designed for a shower or a bath, I created it one winter when I found myself exfoliating less yet still slathering my body with moisturizers and oils to stay hydrated. In the winter months, it's easy to forget to exfoliate, but it's necessary for maintaining a healthy glow, especially when moisturizing more heavily. I love this scrub because it smells cozy and the cinnamon and essential oils promote circulation and warmth in the skin. Plus, it leaves you smelling delicious and can be made with things that are already in your kitchen, provided you're a baker.

METHOD

1. In a small bowl, mix together the sugar and cinnamon.
2. Add the apricot kernel oil and essential oils and mix together with a spoon or your hands until fully incorporated.

APPLICATION

1. Starting at the feet, apply the scrub with your hands in small circular motions over the whole body.
2. Once completely covered in the scrub, rinse it off in the shower.
3. Breathe deeply.

STORAGE

Keep away from moisture in an airtight container for up to 2 weeks. Try to avoid water getting in the scrub.

Lavender Sugar Salt Scrub with Love from Grasse, France

A loving scrub for my grandmother.

TIME: 10 minutes

MAKES: 12 ounces (360 mL) scrub

YOU'LL NEED: a small bowl and a 12-ounce (360 mL) container with a lid

COMPONENTS

½ cup fine salt

½ cup organic white sugar

½ cup organic virgin olive oil

20 drops lavender essential oil

Simplicity at its finest—this sugar and salt scrub is made with olive oil and is inspired by the south of France, where lavender fields and olive oil are plenty. I fell in love with the aroma of lavender at age 10 because my grandmother used a French lavender hand and foot cream. She was my favourite person in the world, so naturally the aroma will forever be associated with her and my memories of her.

I use this scrub when I need a little reminder of the beauty of family. In true French fashion, I could have created the scrub with a stick of butter (which you absolutely could do, by the way), but I prefer a healthier and dairy-free option using olive oil. I hope this calming and wholesome scrub becomes part of your evening bathing routine—complete with white linen towels and a candle burning—in the same way it has very much become a part of mine.

METHOD

1. In a small bowl, mix together the salt and sugar.
2. Add the olive oil and essential oil and mix together with a spoon or your hands until fully incorporated.

APPLICATION

1. Starting at the feet, apply the scrub with your hands in small circular motions over the whole body.
2. Once completely covered in the scrub, rinse it off in the shower.
3. Breathe deeply.

STORAGE

Keep away from moisture in an airtight container for up to 2 weeks. Try to avoid water getting in the scrub.

BATH OILS AND MILKS

Bath oil has been used for hundreds of years and was originally a way for women to scent themselves with perfumes. It not only helps create a hydrating and moisturizing experience, but also leaves the skin hydrated and smelling beautiful in a subtle way (even sometimes the morning after). These simple recipes create products that are similar to body oils but contain less carrier oil and more aroma. I like using them on a Sunday evening with my bath or on the night before an important event, so that I have a base layer of nourished and sweet-smelling skin to take me into the next day. It's a simple evening ritual that takes no extra time and leaves you feeling like you were at the spa. These oils can also be used in an evening foot soak, which is especially lovely during colder winter months for hydrating dry feet.

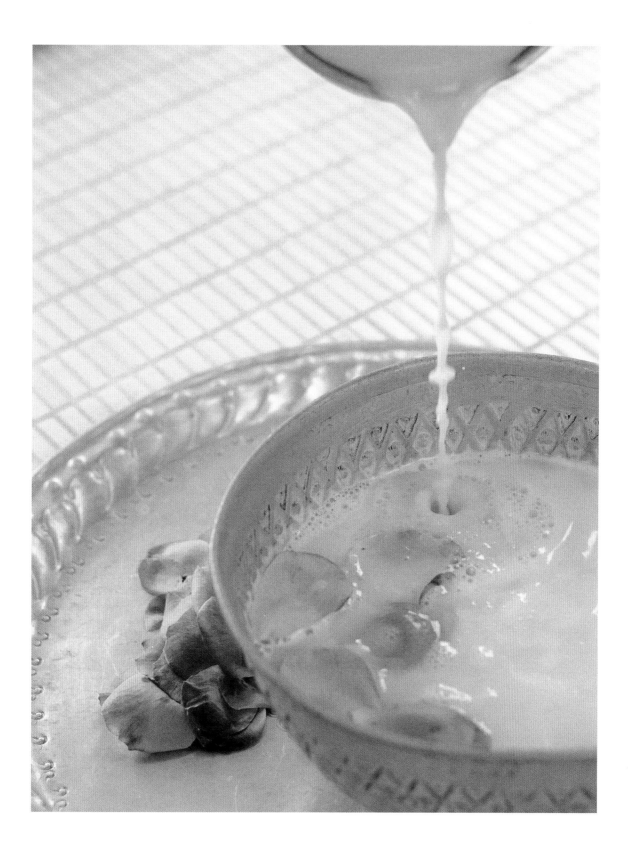

Sweet Dreams Sweet Almond Bath Oil

"Let her sleep, for when she wakes she will move mountains."

TIME: 2 minutes

MAKES: 1 bath oil experience

COMPONENTS

1 tablespoon sweet almond oil

7 drops lavender essential oil

4 drops rosemary essential oil

2 drops cedarwood essential oil

A bath oil is a simple way to integrate the benefits of essential oils into your daily routine. Evening baths got me through the toughest of days while starting our company and are still something I look forward to at the end of a very long, hectic day. Even if I can only fit in a 10-minute bath at 12:10 am, at least I have a small window to soak my body and take some of the load off. I also find that I sleep much better and wake up much more rejuvenated.

In this recipe, I combine some of my favourite relaxation oils. Lavender is one of my favourite bedtime scents and when paired with cedarwood, it helps ground the body and calm a busy mind. Rosemary is thought to help with memory and even with remembering dreams when inhaled before bed. I hope this bath oil provides you with as much relaxation as it has provided me.

METHOD

1. Draw a warm bath. Add all the oils when the bath is full and you are just about to get in.

APPLICATION

1. Soak in the bath for at least 15 minutes.
2. Use your hands to rub any oil sitting on the surface of the water into the skin.

Coconut Milk and Honey Bath Soak

Because who doesn't want to bathe in coconut milk?

TIME: 10 minutes

MAKES: 1 milk bath experience

COMPONENTS

1 cup organic canned full-fat coconut milk

2 tablespoons organic liquid honey

10 drops lavender essential oil

5 drops cedarwood essential oil

5 drops geranium essential oil

Using a dairy-free milk that has a high percentage of moisturizing fats is a calming and soothing way to nourish the skin in the bath. Plus, the sweet aroma adds another layer of relaxation to a simple evening bath experience. Coconut milk is something easy to pick up on your next trip to the grocery store. I always keep a few cans in my kitchen—not for cooking but for when I need a soothing coconut milk bath.

METHOD

1. Draw a warm bath. Add the coconut milk, honey and essential oils when the bath is full and you are just about to get in.

APPLICATION

1. Soak in the bath for as long as you need.
2. Use your hands to rub any oil sitting on the surface of the water into the skin.

Bath Fizzes

TIME: 30 minutes + overnight
to cure
MAKES: 16 fizz cubes
YOU'LL NEED: a medium bowl,
a flexible ice cube tray and an
airtight container

COMPONENTS

1 cup baking soda

½ cup citric acid

½ cup cornstarch

1 teaspoon water

Your favourite evening bath fizz
blend (see below)

STORAGE

Keep in an airtight container in a
cool, dry place for up to 1
month.

Playing with different ways of bringing aroma into your day is fun when you can experiment with different products and experiences. I love using a fizzing sensation in the bath because it brings freshness and lightness to an evening experience. These bath fizzes can be made in batches for a fun pop of essential oils. You can pair these bath fizzes with bath oils to layer scents and experiences. These little fizz cubes also make a fun DIY gift for friends, especially around the holidays when everyone is busy and in need of a good soak in the bathtub.

METHOD

1. In a medium bowl, combine the baking soda, citric acid and cornstarch.
2. Slowly add the water and essential oils blend and whisk until the mixture achieves a wet sand consistency.
3. Lightly pack the mixture into the compartments of an ice cube tray (I love using ones with cute shapes).
4. Leave the mixture to cure overnight in a dry space away from temperature changes or sunlight.
5. Carefully remove the fizz cubes from the tray and allow them to dry further on a towel for 2 to 4 hours (depending on how humid your climate is).

APPLICATION

1. Draw a warm bath, then add 2 fizz cubes.
2. Soak in the bath for as long as you need. Take some deep breaths as the aroma releases. Stretch your arms upward to allow the lungs to open and improve deep breathing.

Essential Oil Aroma Blends for Evening Bath Fizzes

BRAIN FOG CALM DOWN

A grounding blend designed to fizz away brain fog at the end of a long day.

6 drops cedarwood essential oil

2 drops geranium essential oil

2 drops frankincense essential oil

YOGA IN THE BATH

All things yoga from the comfort of your own bathtub—no stretching required.

5 drops spruce essential oil

3 drops frankincense essential oil

2 drops lemon essential oil

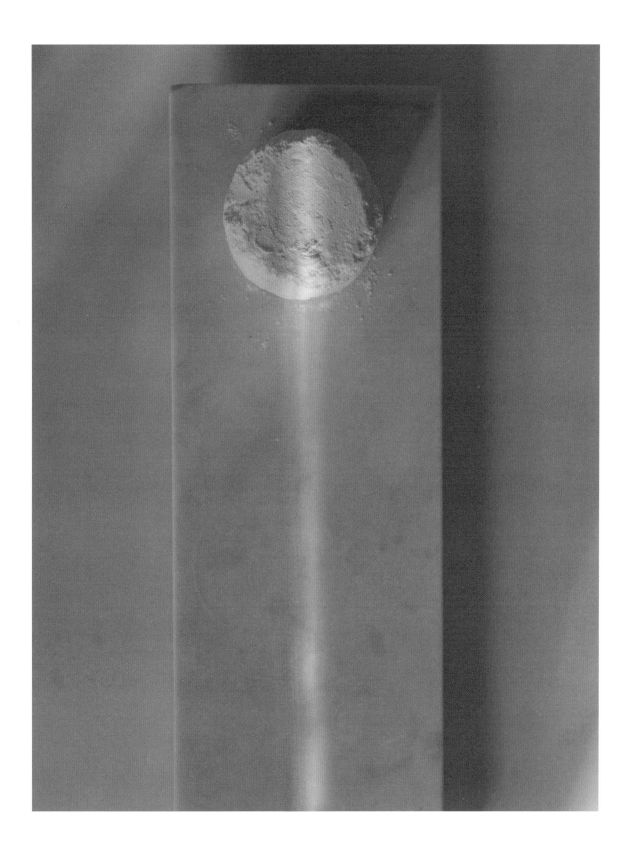

RELAXING EVENING STRETCH

Using aroma strategically at different times in my day has become a practice that really grounds and centres me, especially before bed. I make this mist and keep it in a large mist bottle in my home. Misting it on my yoga mat before an evening stretch is one of my favourite ways to end a day. When I'm travelling, I make a smaller version of this mist to take on the road with me and often mist it onto a towel for my evening stretch when I don't have a yoga mat. I hope this mist and the three simple stretches I've provided create space for you to breathe, reflect and put to rest the business of your day.

RELAXING YOGA MAT MIST

This simple blend is made of eucalyptus essential oil to help promote deep breathing, frankincense essential oil to help ground and create ritual, and lavender essential oil to calm and soothe. Make it in a large batch to use at home or in a small travel-sized batch so you can take the aroma with you.

TIME: 2 minutes
MAKES: 4 ounces (120 mL) mist
YOU'LL NEED: a 4-ounce (120 mL) mist bottle

COMPONENTS

8 tablespoons filtered water (or hydrosol of your choice; I love lavender hydrosol)

5 drops lavender essential oil

3 drops frankincense essential oil

3 drops cedarwood essential oil

2 drops eucalyptus essential oil

METHOD

1. Mix together the water and essential oils in a mist bottle and shake to combine.

APPLICATION

1. Shake gently before each use.
2. Mist over yoga mat and wipe down using a cloth.

STORAGE

Keep in a cool, dry place away from direct sunlight for up to 1 month.

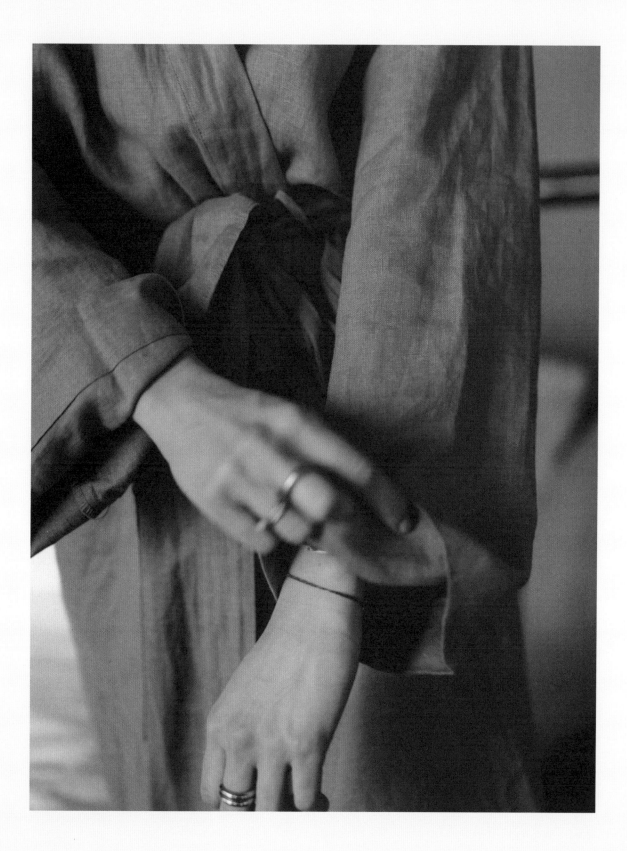

THREE SIMPLE EVENING STRETCHES TO HELP YOU UNWIND

Here are a few simple stretches that you can do on your yoga mat or from the comfort of your bed. I hope they create space for you to breathe, reflect and put to rest the business of your day.

CHILD'S POSE

Sit up straight on your heels with your knees pointing slightly out to the sides. Gently roll your torso forward until your forehead rests on the mat in front of you (adjust the position of your knees for maximum comfort). Lower your chest as close to your knees or the mat as you comfortably can, extending your arms in front of you and stretching your fingers outward with your palms on the mat. Hold the pose for 2 to 4 minutes. Breathe.

LEGS UP THE WALL

Sit facing a wall (or your headboard, if you're in your bed) with your bottom approximately 6 inches away from the wall. Lying on your back, extend your legs up the wall with your feet relaxed in a slightly flexed position. Keep your arms by your sides in a comfortable position, palms facing up. Hold the pose for 1 to 2 minutes. Breathe.

EVENING RITUAL GODDESS STRETCH

Lie on your back with your legs slightly bent and knees angled slightly outward. Touch the soles of your feet together, letting your knees fall open naturally; this will form a butterfly shape. Allow your arms to fall comfortably beside your torso in whatever form or shape is most relaxing. If your knees or hips hurt or feel too strained, place a pillow underneath each knee to take tension off the joints. Hold the pose for 3 to 5 minutes. Breathe.

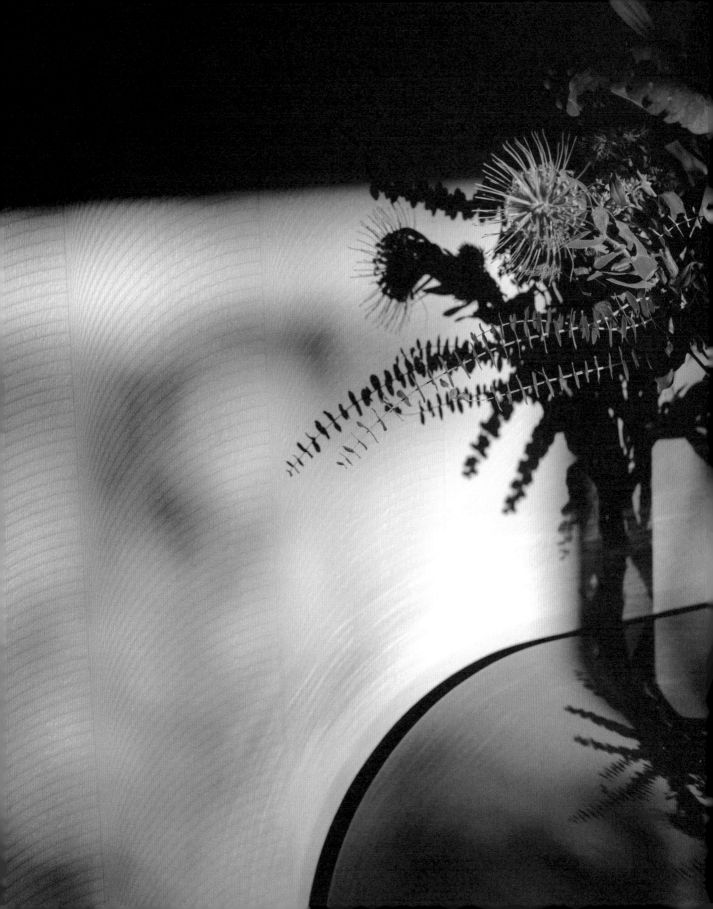

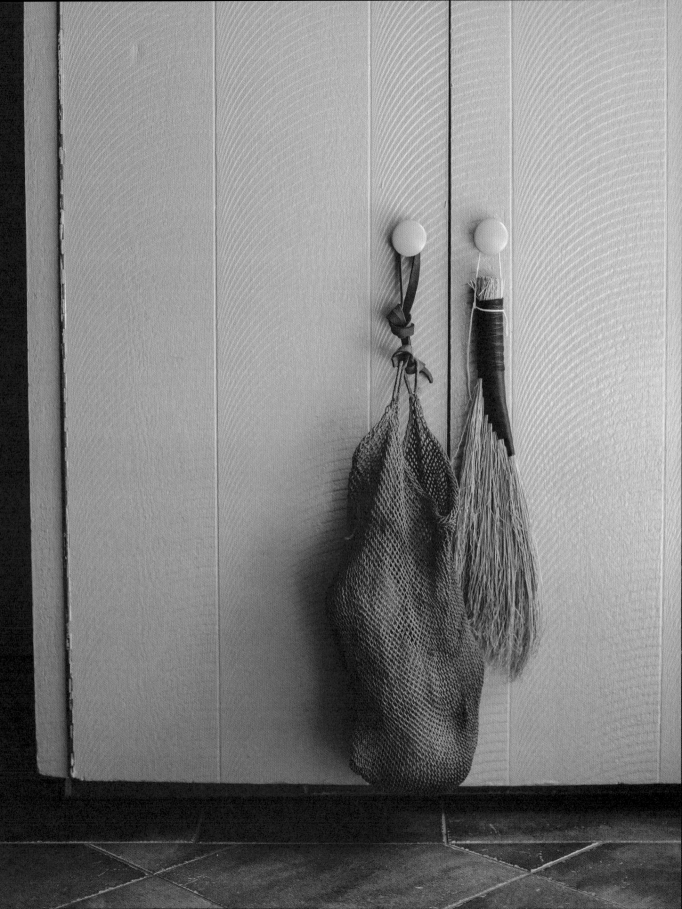

HOME

A beautiful and often unnoticed sensation happens when you smell "home"—whether that's the aroma of where you grew up, an apartment that holds happy memories, or your current home. It's an unconscious recognition, and it makes that familiar space feel like home, whatever that means to you. There's a science and an art to scenting a space, and this juxtaposition has fascinated me since starting my wellness company. Using scent to cue the brain to realize that a space means something is an incredibly powerful concept. For instance, lavender in a bedroom calms and creates a sense of peace and lightness, while grapefruit in a kitchen feels fresh, bold and crisp. Eucalyptus in the bathroom brings a sense of cleanliness, order and vitality to my morning shower or makes me feel rejuvenated, awake and connected to nature during my evening bath. These are all feelings and moods that inspire me through the unconscious influence of scent.

Cueing our brain to get into these states through aroma is the ultimate way to schedule our days and shift our focus and intentions in the most understated yet dramatic way. Nomadic tribes use aroma by burning herbs and wood when they reach a new camp—a ritual that is the essence of scenting your home . . . or rather, making a home through scent. I've used essential oils as a means to explore a way of living with intention though aroma and, in doing so, a natural way of living. Not only do they create a beautiful way to play with scent and create moods and intentions in a space, but their chemical properties make them useful in the home in many other ways—in how we clean, deodorize and live in our home.

This section is very dear to my heart because it shares some of the simple ways we can live more closely with nature and its intrinsic properties. My hope for this section is that you will feel a playfulness and a sense of healthy control over your space through the alchemy of mixing and blending. I also hope that these simple recipes will inspire deep thought about the spaces you move through during your day and how their aroma can help you bring out your best self.

DIFFUSER GENERAL
BLENDING GUIDE

For this section, I've put together a general guide for combining essential oils in an ultrasonic diffuser. I want to stress that this is only a guide, and by no means should it be followed perfectly. Scent should be playful and intuitive—there's no need to overthink it. I believe aromas should be blended based on your intuition and your first reaction to a scent, especially when you're just starting out. My goal is for you to experiment with essential oils and create aromas for your living spaces that are as unique and complex as you are.

This simple guide is a great starting point to help you learn how to blend essential oil aromas for your home diffuser. There are a few ways of blending essential oils, and one way to begin is by using a technique I learned in Grasse, France (the perfume capital of the world). They have been making perfume there for hundreds of years, and most fashion labels still have their head "nose" or perfume maker there to sample botanical extracts and scent combinations.

In general, a great rule of thumb for blending different families of essential oils together is:

Citrus + Herbal
Floral + Woodsy

To make a diffuser aroma using this traditional technique, you blend essential oils according to notes (top, middle and base notes). Each note is determined by the order in which it "comes off the notes" or, in more simple terms, the order in which you smell it. In perfume making, you smell a top note first, followed by a middle note and then the base note, which is more likely to linger on the skin and evolve as time passes.

A traditionally made perfume or home aroma is usually made up of three parts top note, two parts middle note and one part base note. The base note is usually added in smaller proportions because it has a stronger and more prominent aroma. Using traditional perfume blending techniques for your home diffuser blends will result in unique and complex aromas that guests will be inspired and intrigued by, not to mention that there is something really old world about the whole experience. Examples of each "notes" are included on the opposite page.

TOP NOTES

Evaporate off the nose first, fading quickly after being the first aroma the nose experiences.

Anise
Basil
Bergamot
Grapefruit

Spearmint
Sweet orange
Tangerine
Tea tree

MIDDLE NOTES

Linger slightly longer and hold together the top and base notes.

Cardamom
Clary sage
Cypress
Eucalyptus
Geranium
Ginger
Juniper berry

Lavender
Palmarosa
Pine
Roman chamomile
Rosemary
Spruce

BASE NOTES

The base of the aroma, a deeper scent that keeps the aroma on the skin or in the air the longest and grounds the entire aroma.

Frankincense
Jasmine
Myrrh
Patchouli
Rose

Sandalwood
Turmeric
Vanilla
Vetiver
Ylang ylang

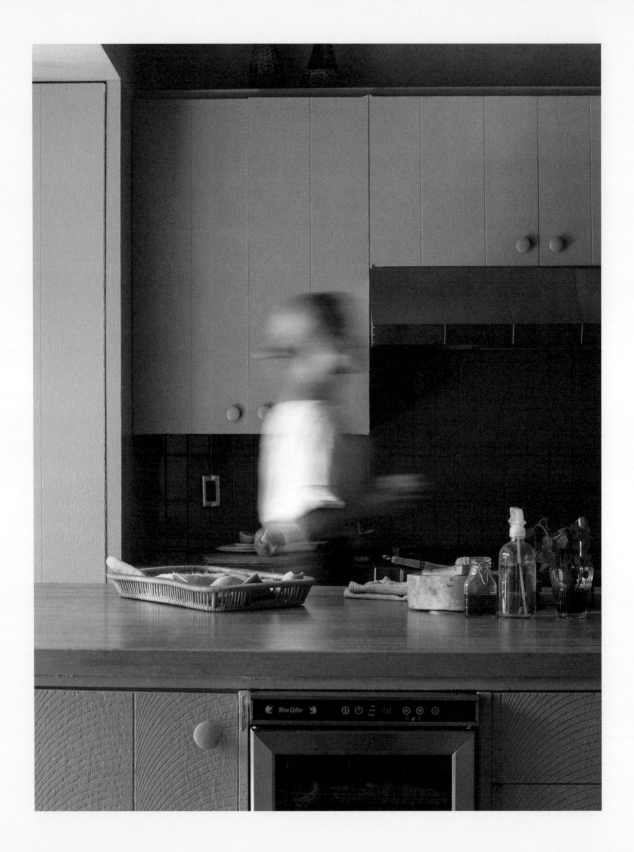

KITCHEN

The kitchen is one of my favourite places to use essential oils because they provide a nice cleaning alternative that is chemical-free. Plus, they smell amazing and add to a cozy kitchen vibe. I'm not a cook, but I make enough of a mess to know that having a simple stash of the perfect essential oils for cleanup is a bright and fresh way to bring a new level of cleanliness to your kitchen.

ESSENTIAL OILS FOR THE KITCHEN

SWEET ORANGE ESSENTIAL OIL

Sweet orange essential oil is an easy, multi-purpose essential oil that helps naturally cut grease from pots and pans or your stove. I keep it by my sink and add it to dishwater for a little extra kick during cleanup time.

LEMON ESSENTIAL OIL

There is nothing that smells as clean as lemon. Lemon essential oil is created by cold pressing lemon rinds and extracting the oil from them. While it might sound easy, it takes a lot of lemons to make just a little bottle of essential oil. The potent cleaning factors of the rind are similar to those in sweet orange, and they help naturally cut grease. Lemon is also a healthy way to rinse produce—simply add 5 drops to a large bowl of water, rinse your produce and let dry.

TEA TREE ESSENTIAL OIL

Tea tree essential oil is a great way to naturally clean and disinfect your kitchen surfaces, especially your fridge and sink . . . oh, and those dishcloths that might be smelling less than fresh. It's a must-have in my kitchen because of its naturally antimicrobial and antibacterial properties. I'll usually add a few drops to my dishcloth to wipe down surfaces like kitchen counters before and after food prep.

Countertop Sprays

TIME: 2 minutes

MAKES: 10 ounces (300 mL) countertop spray

YOU'LL NEED: a 12-ounce (360 mL) spray bottle and a funnel (optional)

COMPONENTS

1 cup filtered water

4 tablespoons white vinegar

Your favourite countertop spray blend (see below)

I love making my own simple countertop spray with essential oils—not just because it's more cost effective, but also because it's a lovely way to incorporate a non-toxic alternative to your cleaning routine while also making your own custom kitchen scent. The formula is super simple, and I like making these sprays in small batches so that I can switch up their aroma.

METHOD

1. Using a funnel, add all components to a spray bottle and shake gently to combine.

APPLICATION

1. Shake gently before each use.
2. Mist onto countertop and wipe clean.

STORAGE

Keep in a cool, dry place away from direct sunlight for up to 2 months.

Essential Oil Aroma Blends for Countertop Sprays

CITRUS COUNTERTOP SPRAY

A fresh and bright aroma that makes the kitchen a happy place.

20 drops sweet orange essential oil

5 drops lemongrass essential oil

5 drops peppermint essential oil

HERBAL FRESH COUNTERTOP SPRAY

A perfectly balanced aroma with double the cleaning power.

20 drops grapefruit essential oil

10 drops tea tree essential oil

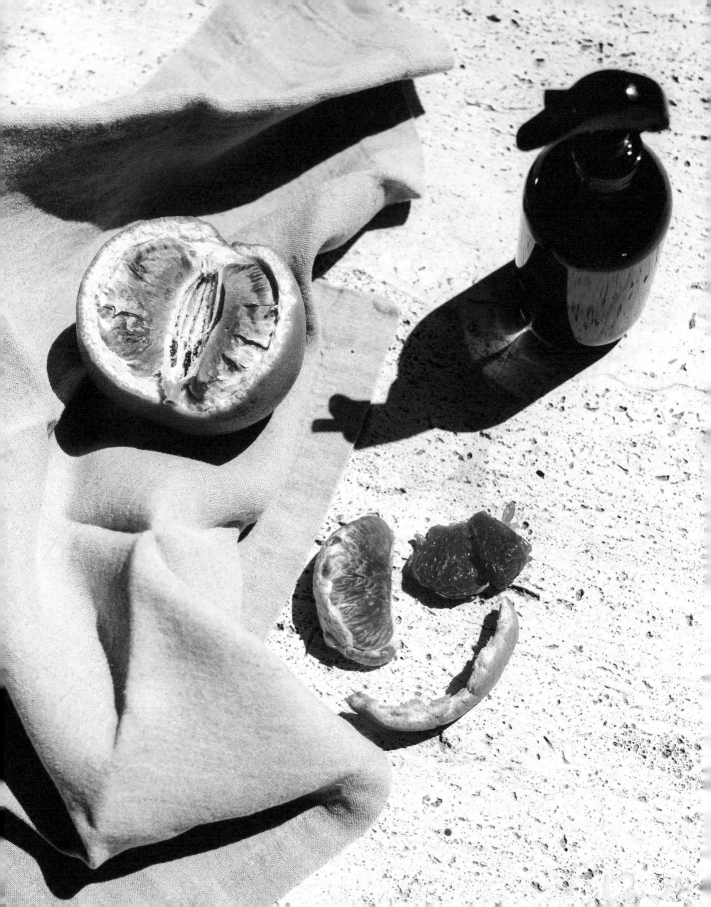

DEODORIZERS

A homemade deodorizer is a super-simple way to keep things smelling fresh, especially in the fridge, garbage and compost areas of your kitchen. These places often are hard to keep smelling good and shouldn't have chemicals and toxic materials around them. Natural deodorizers are an easy fix for scenting some of the not-so-lovely spaces of your home without using chemicals. They use baking soda, which I love because it's completely natural and affordable, which means sprinkling it in your garbage can is easy to do. I create the following recipes at different intervals throughout the month to maintain freshness throughout my kitchen.

Fridge Freshener

Keep your fridge smelling as fresh as the bunches of kale in it.

When I open my fridge, I want it to smell fresh and crisp. Produce and leftovers can leave the fridge smelling like none of these things, so I started creating this fridge deodorizer that I try to switch up every 2 to 4 weeks. This deodorizer is especially helpful in office fridges, where things tend to get pretty messy and stinky quite quickly.

TIME: 3 minutes

MAKES: 8.45 ounces (250 mL) deodorizer

YOU'LL NEED: a mason jar or ceramic tray

COMPONENTS

1 cup baking soda

10 drops peppermint essential oil

10 drops tea tree essential oil

5 drops grapefruit essential oil

5 drops sweet orange essential oil

STORAGE

Keep in the fridge. Replace every 2 to 4 weeks, depending on freshness.

METHOD

1. Add the baking soda to a mason jar or ceramic tray.
2. Add all the essential oils, then mix with a spoon, trying to break up clumps of essential oil as best as possible.

APPLICATION

1. Put the freshener in the fridge door or the back of the fridge.
2. Stir once a week or do a quick top up of essential oils, adding 2 drops peppermint, 2 drops tea tree, 1 drop grapefruit and 1 drop sweet orange to keep it smelling extra fresh.

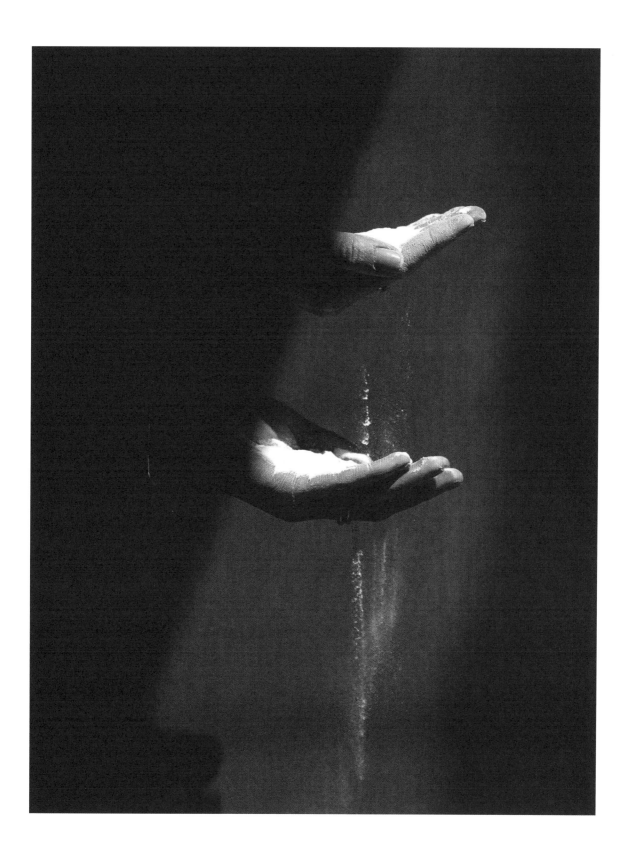

Trash Can Deodorizer

Proof that taking out the garbage doesn't have to be scary.

TIME: 1 minute

MAKES: 8.45 ounces (250 mL) deodorizer

YOU'LL NEED: a small bowl, a spoon and 1 sheet paper towel or newspaper

COMPONENTS

1 cup baking soda

10 drops tea tree essential oil

10 drops spruce essential oil

5 drops lemon essential oil

5 drops lemongrass essential oil

An incredibly simple way to make taking out the trash just slightly more bearable is by adding this essential oil mixture to the base of your garbage can. This is a little secret I started a few years ago, and it means that when I pull the bag out of the garbage can, it's so much more pleasant. While you're cooking, your trash can is usually opening and closing a lot—this is a super-simple way to not let that odour take over your kitchen. Plus, guests will be greeted by a nice smell if they're helping you prep.

METHOD

1. Add the baking soda to a small bowl.
2. Add all the essential oils, then mix with a spoon, trying to break up clumps of essential oil as best as possible.

APPLICATION

1. Line the bottom of the garbage can with a sheet of paper towel or newspaper.
2. Sprinkle a thin layer of deodorizer over the paper towel or newspaper, about ¼ cup.
3. Top up essential oils by adding 2 drops tea tree, 2 drops spruce, 1 drop lemon and 1 drop lemongrass to the deodorizer whenever you need it to be fresher between garbage bag changes.

STORAGE

Keep at the bottom of your trash can. Replace every 1 to 2 weeks, depending on freshness.

Compost Deodorizer

Good for the earth and good for you, too.

TIME: 5 minutes

MAKES: 8.45 ounces (250 mL) deodorizer

YOU'LL NEED: a small bowl or mason jar

COMPONENTS

1 cup baking soda

10 drops tea tree essential oil

10 drops cedarwood essential oil

10 drops spruce essential oil

Composting in the city is so very different from the experience I had growing up in a rural area. We had a large outdoor composting station in our backyard that produced the most beautiful and dark dirt rich with nutrients. My parents would add this dirt to their vegetable gardens in the backyard, which resulted in yields of lettuce, garlic, peas, strawberries, kale, carrots and potatoes all summer long. Composting food scraps is never seamless in an apartment or office, and while I'm always trying my best, any way to keep the process smelling and looking cleaner and more organized is always a little win in living more naturally.

METHOD

1. Add the baking soda to a small bowl or mason jar.
2. Add all the essential oils, then mix with a spoon, trying to break up clumps of essential oil as best as possible.

APPLICATION

1. Sprinkle ¼ cup deodorizer directly into your compost bin to help absorb any unpleasant aroma from the compost.
2. You can also use tea tree essential oil to rinse out your compost container when you are emptying it to help kill bacteria and leave it smelling fresh.

STORAGE

Keep near your compost bin. Replace every 5 to 7 days, depending on freshness.

SINK AND DISH CLEANERS

Time spent at the sink is never my favourite part of the day, but there is something satisfying about a sparkling clean kitchen sink. The natural antibacterial properties of essential oils and their ability to break down food grease make them necessary to have beside my kitchen sink. Sweet orange essential oil, peppermint essential oil, lemon essential oil and tea tree essential oil are my go-to oils, and they have become something I use every day for a little germ-fighting boost. Here are three quick tips that will result in less bacteria, a fresh-smelling sink and a more positive kitchen cleaning experience all around.

QUICK TIP #1: CITRUS DISH SOAP

To naturally increase the cleaning power of my dish soap, I add essential oils like lemon, eucalyptus, sweet orange, tea tree and lavender to my dishwater. They're known to have antibacterial properties, and just 10 to 15 drops of any of these essential oils in the sink helps elevate the experience of dishwashing. Adding a citrus oil to dishwater is especially helpful because the oil's properties naturally break down grease. I add 10 drops of organic sweet orange essential oil to my dishwater each night—it helps clean pots and pans, and the aroma transforms the chore of washing dishes into something that actually puts me in a good mood.

QUICK TIP #2: SWEET AND HERBAL SINK SCRUB

This is a super-easy, natural sink scrub that will leave your sink (especially if it's stainless steel) looking really beautiful and shiny and, of course, smelling amazing. All you have to do is sprinkle ¼ cup of baking soda into the sink and add 10 to 15 drops of essential oils—my favourites are tea tree, sweet orange and peppermint. The texture of the baking soda helps polish the stainless steel and remove stains and dirt, while the essential oils help kill bacteria. Scrub using a wire brush or a dishcloth and rinse away any baking soda residue to leave your sink with a fresh, clean finish.

QUICK TIP #3: DISHCLOTH DISINFECTANT

Keep your dishcloth clean between uses by rinsing it with hot water, adding 10 drops of tea tree essential oil to it and then giving it one last rinse before ringing it out to dry. The tea tree essential oil has been known to have antimicrobial and antibacterial properties, meaning it's great for keeping dishcloths at their freshest.

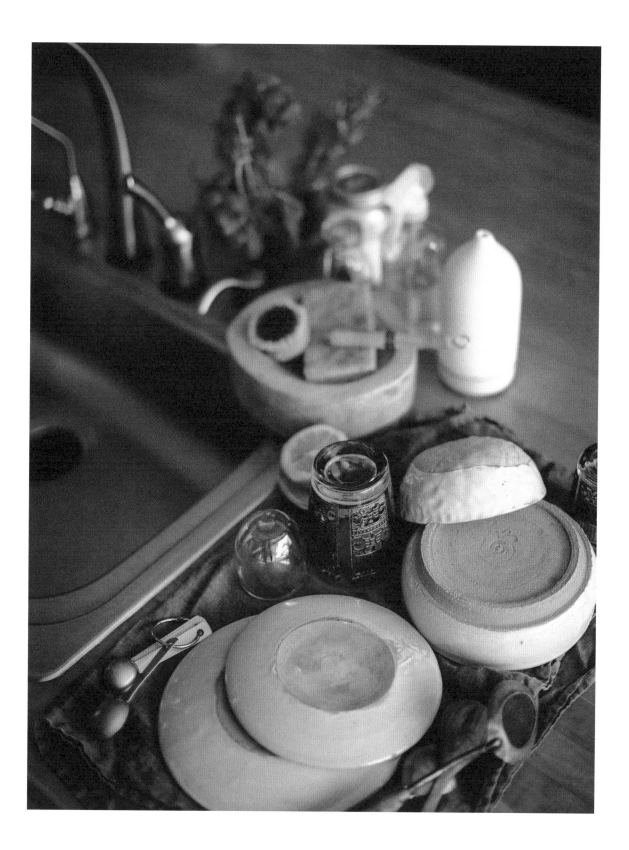

KITCHEN DIFFUSER BLENDS

These blends are great to use in the kitchen on weekends to freshen things up. They've become a staple ritual in my cooking prep (especially when I'm about to cook with garlic or onions). Before I start cooking, I add one of these blends to my diffuser in the kitchen and turn it on—it keeps things smelling fresh and clean, regardless of the absolute mess I'm making on my stove and countertop.

So Fresh and So Clean

A blend that gives off ultra-fresh vibes at any hour of the day.

10 drops spruce essential oil

10 drops grapefruit essential oil

The Lazy Housekeeper

A blend that makes it smell like you just cleaned your house, even when you didn't.

5 drops tea tree essential oil

5 drops lemon essential oil

5 drops peppermint essential oil

4 drops sweet orange essential oil

3 drops spruce essential oil

Citrus Fruit Salad

A blend that smells like you just peeled and plated a giant fresh citrus fruit salad.

7 drops grapefruit essential oil

5 drops sweet orange essential oil

5 drops lemon essential oil

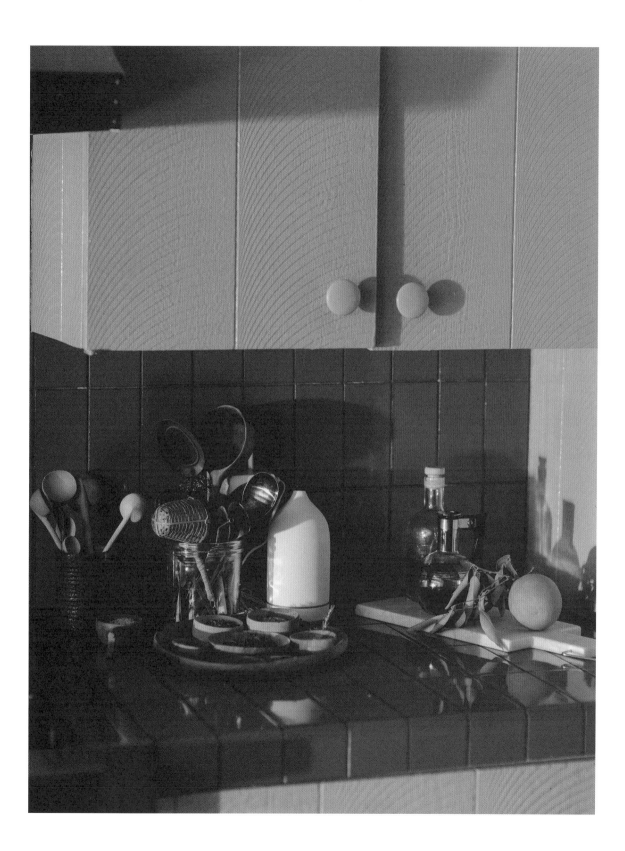

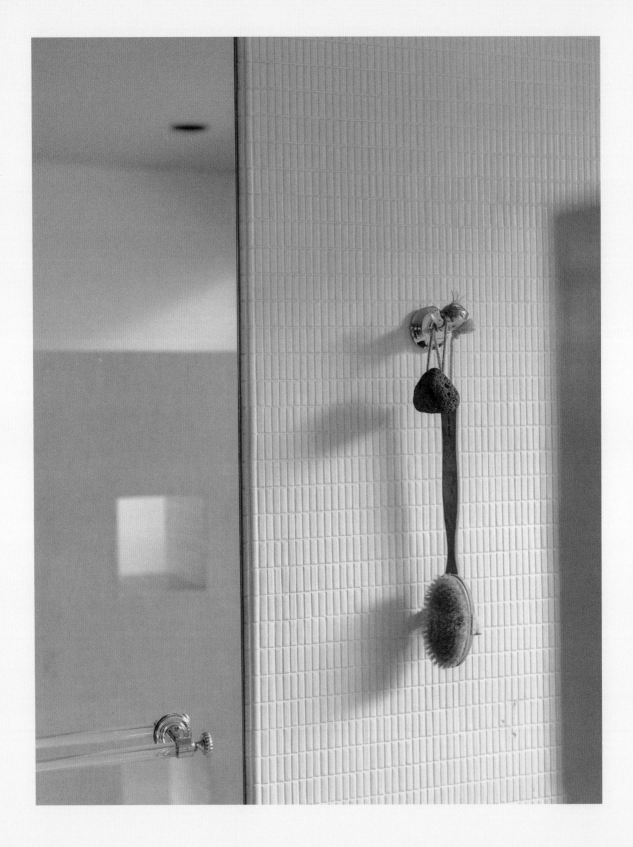

BATHROOM

Many of the products made from the recipes in the beauty and body sections of this book are used in a bathroom. Body scrubs, bathing, face and hair masks and dry brushing are all ancient acts of self-care and wellness that help get us out of our heads and reacquainted with our bodies. Creating a serene space in your bathroom can turn an everyday chore into a beautiful ritual. Adding some pieces of art or products that are special to you to your bathroom can help turn it into an oasis, and cleaning your bathroom with essential oils is an effective and easy way to keep it smelling and feeling like a spa. Using all-natural cleaning products is important, and it's even more important in the shower and bath, where you are submerging your skin.

ESSENTIAL OILS FOR THE BATHROOM

EUCALYPTUS

Nothing smells more like a spa than eucalyptus essential oil. It is readily used in spa steam rooms and showers because it helps cue the body to take full, deep breaths. It also has natural antibacterial and antimicrobial properties, which make it helpful for keeping showers and bathtubs clean in a completely natural way. There is a bottle of eucalyptus essential oil in my shower at all times and another bottle under my sink for cleaning purposes.

GERANIUM

This beautiful floral essential oil has slightly minty undertones. I love adding it to bathroom cleaning products because it adds a floral dimension that makes the space feel more like an oasis. Geranium essential oil is lovely to add to a bathtub cleaner because anything left over as residue just makes your bath smell amazing. It's balancing for the skin and mind and is also used in a number of skincare oils, which makes it a bathroom essential.

PEPPERMINT

Ultra fresh and associated with that minty-fresh feeling of toothpaste and mouthwash, peppermint essential oil has the same tingling sensation and aroma. With natural antibacterial and antimicrobial properties, it's a bathroom staple. I keep one bottle of peppermint essential oil beside my toothbrush to help disinfect it naturally between brushings, and I also keep a bottle in the cabinet under my sink to use in cleaning products.

Bathtub Scrub

A simple scrub that keeps things natural.

TIME: 2 minutes

MAKES: 8.45 ounces (250 mL) scrub

YOU'LL NEED: a small bowl or mason jar, a spoon and a scrub brush or cloth

COMPONENTS

1 cup baking soda

15 drops eucalyptus essential oil

15 drops peppermint essential oil

10 drops geranium essential oil

This scrub can be used in your toilet or bathtub and makes it easy to remove residue, stains and grime left over from showers and baths. Compared to the more toxic bathtub and shower cleaners, this one is a natural, refreshing alternative. You don't even need gloves to apply it.

METHOD

1. Mix together all components in a bowl or jar, using a spoon to break up clumps of essential oils as best as possible.

APPLICATION

1. Sprinkle ¼ to ½ cup at a time over the bottom of the bathtub, then add a thin layer of warm water to the bathtub.
2. Using a scrub brush or cloth, scrub the bathtub.
3. Add more warm water and continue scrubbing.
4. When the bathtub feels clean, rinse with very warm water.

STORAGE

Keep leftover scrub in an airtight container for up to 1 month. Use it between showers to keep the shower fresh.

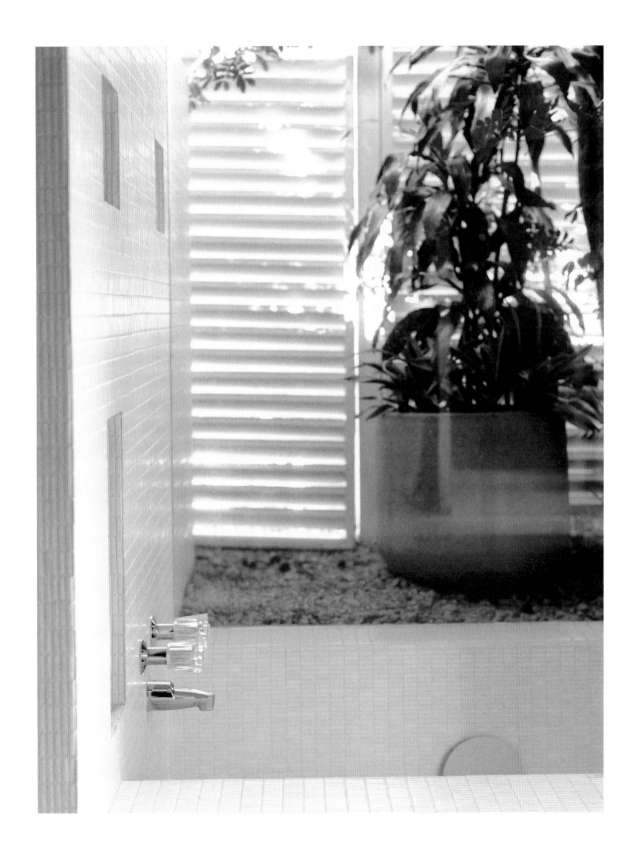

Shower Cleaning Spray

Your new shower saviour.

TIME: 5 minutes

MAKES: 16 ounces (480 mL) shower spray

YOU'LL NEED: a 16-ounce (480 mL) spray bottle

COMPONENTS

1¾ cup filtered water

¼ cup white vinegar

30 drops tea tree essential oil

20 drops peppermint essential oil

20 drops grapefruit essential oil

10 drops eucalyptus essential oil

I'm passionate about simplifying cleaning and other tasks, and I am an advocate of doing things in the moment that will save me time in the future. I try to build cleaning tasks into my everyday routine to save me time, so that on weekends and evenings I can focus on spending time with people I really care about. I've created this shower cleaning spray, which I keep in my shower and mist my shower and bathtub with after each use. The antibacterial properties of the essential oils and vinegar kill any germs or mildew that might start growing and prevent the need for more thorough cleanings.

METHOD
1. Add all components to a spray bottle.
2. Gently shake to combine components.

APPLICATION
1. Spray the shower and bathtub after each use.
2. Spray the inside of the shower curtain or shower liner to prevent mildew.

STORAGE
Keep in a cool, dry place for 6 months to 1 year.

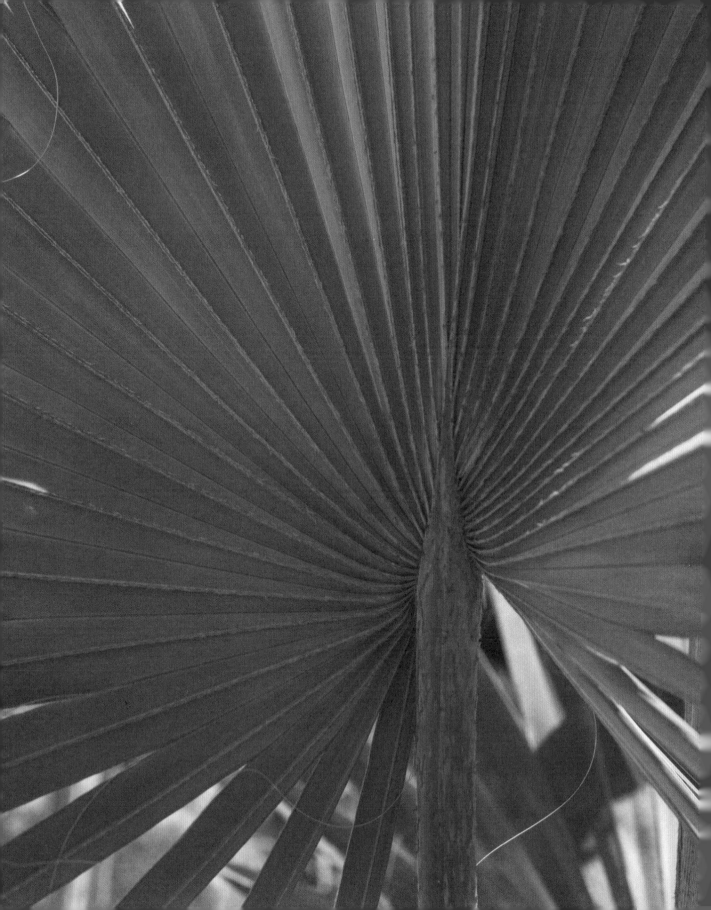

Towel Spray

Better than monogramming.

TIME: 2 minutes

MAKES: 16 ounces (480 mL) towel spray

YOU'LL NEED: a 16-ounce (480 mL) spray bottle

COMPONENTS

2 cups filtered water

20 drops cedarwood essential oil

20 drops bergamot essential oil

7 drops eucalyptus essential oil

Scented towels feel so luxurious, but they are so simple to have and are an easy everyday luxury you can incorporate into your routine before you get in the shower. I make a new towel spray seasonally, and creating a custom towel aroma is a fun way to make your guests feel even more special in your home. Try spraying your bedsheets, too.

METHOD

1. Combine all components in a spray bottle with a fine mist setting.

APPLICATION

1. Shake gently before each use.
2. Mist towels liberally before getting in the shower.

STORAGE

Keep in a cool, dry place (like your linen closet) for up to 2 months.

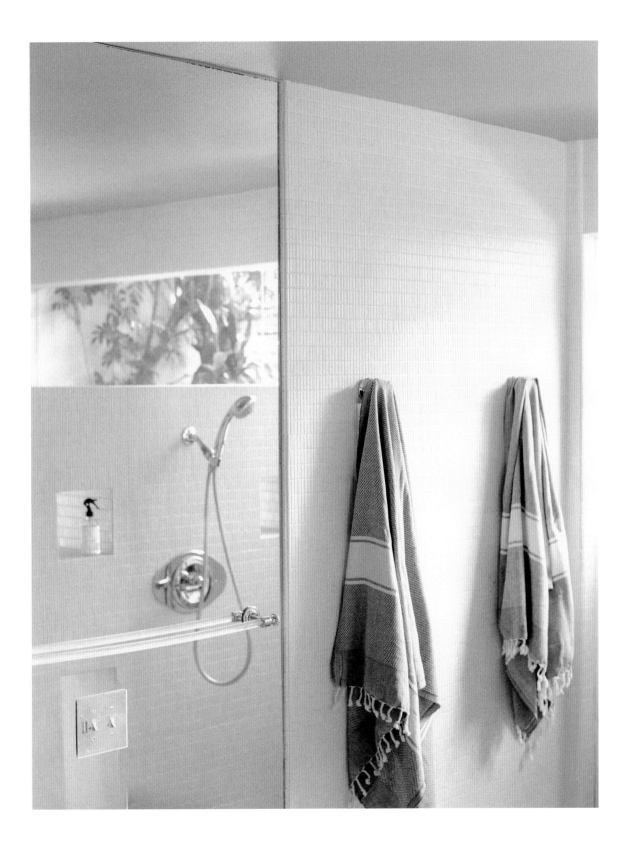

Toilet Deodorizer

An on-the-go blend to leave things smelling fresh.

TIME: 2 minutes

MAKES: 0.67 ounce (20 mL) deodorizer

YOU'LL NEED: a 1-ounce (30 mL) dropper bottle

COMPONENTS

4 teaspoons sweet almond oil

30 drops ylang ylang essential oil

30 drops peppermint essential oil

10 drops tea tree essential oil

5 drops bergamot essential oil

This little bottle of deodorizer can live by your toilet (or even in your purse) for those moments when you find yourself wanting to leave the bathroom smelling better than you found it. This toilet deodorizer comes in handy after using the washroom and leaves the toilet smelling literally like flowers.

METHOD

1. Mix all components in a dropper bottle.

APPLICATION

1. Add 5 to 10 drops of deodorizer to a toilet as needed (it will leave a small film of oil on the surface of the water). To make it extra fresh, flush the toilet and the splashing of the water will intensify the aroma of the essential oils.

STORAGE

Keep in a cool, dry place for up to 2 months.

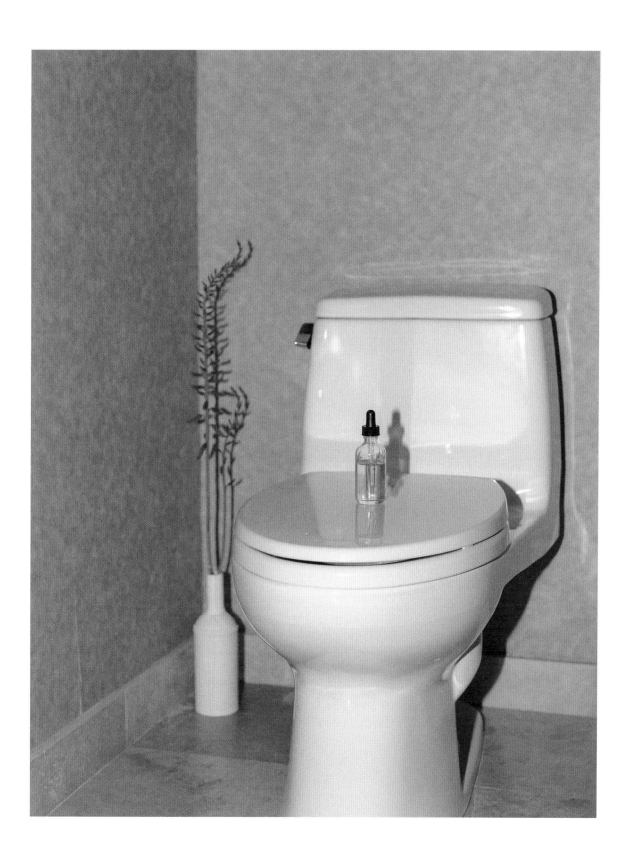

DIY SAUNA

Saunas and baths are some of the most ancient rituals and practices around self-care and wellness. Ancient Roman texts reference the bath houses as ritualistic places of conversation and community where Romans would bathe in herbs and soaps that held special meaning. Today, saunas, spas and steam rooms still act as sites of cleansing and detoxifying that can be as purging for the mind as for our skin. If you have a sauna in your home, try adding 5 to 10 drops of eucalyptus essential oil and 5 to 10 drops of cedarwood essential oil to the hot rocks. If you don't have a sauna in your home (like most people), I love using face steams and warm baths as excuses to steam up the bathroom, then add some essential oils and take deep breaths.

BELLY BREATHING IN A SAUNA OR WARM BATH

With each deep inhale through the nose, envision a warm yellow light (or whatever colour you associate with kind energy and potential). Envision that light as breath filling your lungs. Using belly breathing, push your lower abdomen out with the inhale, helping to lower the diaphragm and further increase lung capacity. At the top of the inhale, hold the breath for 3 seconds.

On the exhale, envision a grey light (or whatever colour you associate with stale energy) and push that out through your mouth for a count of 5 seconds.

Repeat this pattern three times. I use this technique in the shower and while doing face steams, warm baths or saunas. While the body and skin are detoxifying from the heat of the steam, it's a really beautiful time to envision letting go of stale thoughts and energy that no longer serve you.

I hope this ritual becomes as much of a key cleansing practice in your week as it has been for me. It doesn't need to take place in a fancy sauna. I've practiced belly breathing in a number of places: hotels, planes, boardrooms. It's the practice of the breath and the visual of the light that makes this ritual so cleansing—it's not about waiting for the perfect surroundings.

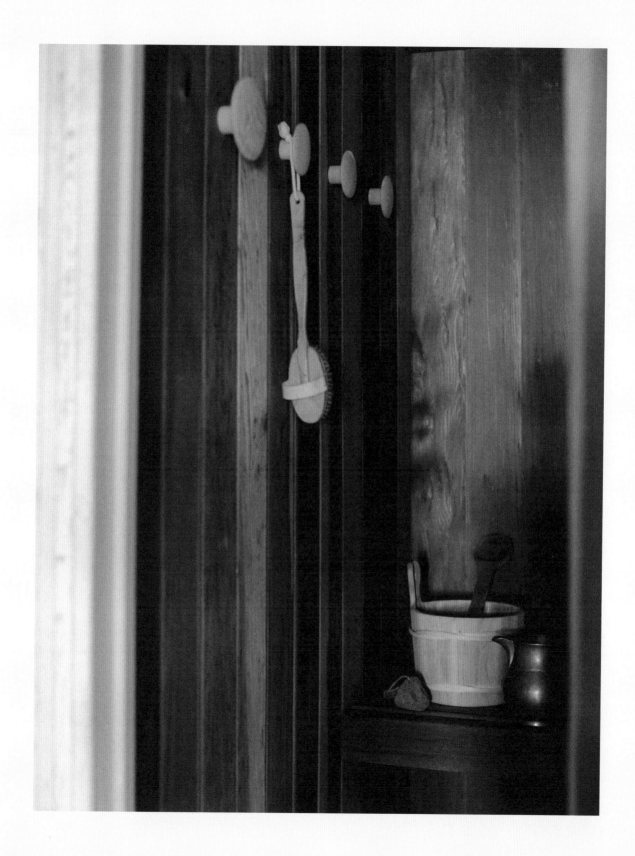

BATHROOM DIFFUSER BLENDS

Diffuser blends that I love for the bathroom depend on the time of day I am using them. What makes a diffuser more adaptable than a candle for the bathroom is that you can set the mood or create an oasis even before you enter the space. Each of these diffuser blends was designed for a specific bathroom ritual, and each one plays with the senses at different times of day and in different routines. Add one of these bathroom blends to an ultrasonic diffuser.

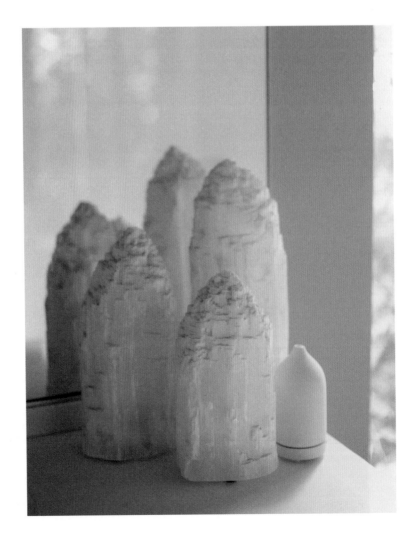

Wake Up, Sleepyhead

A blend that fills your bathroom with the smell of a hundred peeled oranges.

Using citrus aromas in the morning is a subtle way to influence the brain and cue it to wake up naturally. Part of my morning routine involves drinking water as soon as I wake up and turning on my bathroom diffuser with this citrus and herbal blend before I make my matcha.

10 drops sweet orange essential oil

5 drops grapefruit essential oil

2 drops lemon essential oil

Morning Spa Session

A blend that sneaks an early spa moment into your day.

This diffuser blend helps you turn your bathroom into a full-on spa in the morning. No one needs to know that your 5-minute shower smells like a five-star hotel eucalyptus steam room.

10 drops eucalyptus essential oil

3 drops geranium essential oil

2 drops tea tree essential oil

Glowing Girl

A perfect blend to set the mood for a little "you" time.

This is a diffuser blend for late-night bath moments spent with the lights off and the diffuser on. This mix of resinous essential oils combined with floral undertones helps create a sense of ritual and habit that has me craving evening baths as a floral-scented place of serenity.

7 drops ylang ylang essential oil

5 drops frankincense essential oil

5 drops cedarwood essential oil

2 drops bergamot essential oil

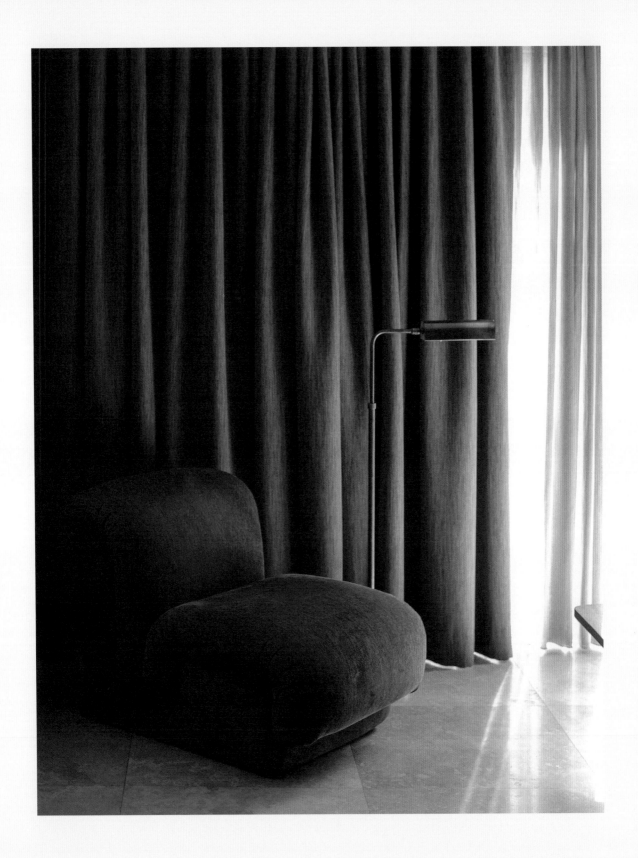

LIVING ROOM

My living room is for reading and for objects that remind me of fond memories. It's a place where some of my favourite art, as well as photographs of family and friends, hang on the walls. Living rooms are also for kids, movie watching, fort building, couch surfing and everything in between. In my opinion, time spent in a living room is time with wine, tea, popcorn, puzzles, magazines and custom-made aromas that tie memories and the ceremony of unwinding into one safe, cozy space.

ESSENTIAL OILS FOR THE LIVING ROOM

BERGAMOT
Bergamot is a citrus essential oil with a spicy aroma—it's the smell and taste that's prominent in Earl Grey tea. It's a very sophisticated citrus aroma with more complexity and depth than any other citrus fruit. Its popularity and prestige means that bergamot essential oil is found in about half of women's perfumes and a third of men's colognes. It's a great multi-use essential oil for the home, and I love it because it's both fresh and comforting.

SPRUCE
Spruce essential oil has a peppery scent that makes it smell slightly lemon-like yet spicy. I love spruce for the living room any time of the year. It pairs beautifully with citrus to feel more uplifting in the warm summer months and can also be used alone or with other deep woodsy aromas to establish a grounded energy during winter.

CEDARWOOD
The scent of a log cabin or cedar sauna wherever you are—cedarwood essential oil brings the grounded energy of wood to your space. Especially with city living, my nose sometimes craves the aroma of nature and trees.

Carpet Deodorizer

A natural approach to tackling those hidden smells.

TIME: 20 minutes

MAKES: 8.45 ounces (250 mL) deodorizer

YOU'LL NEED: a small bowl and a spoon

COMPONENTS

1 cup baking soda

30 drops cedarwood essential oil

20 drops eucalyptus essential oil

10 drops lemon essential oil

I have a lovely dog named Charlie, and she goes everywhere with me, including to the beach almost every day after work (or when we can). She chases seagulls like it's her full-time job and, in the process, gets covered in sand, saltwater and dirt. Having a wet dog in the house more days than not means that every once in a while (or once a week) I love to deodorize my rugs and carpets—especially the rug under my dining room table, where Charlie loves to hide along with a few rogue crumbs.

Carpet and rug deodorizers are often filled with chemicals and preservatives that can be harmful to your pets and irritating to the feet, which is not something I would ever want in a home. Using a natural carpet deodorizer is a simple and effective way to seal a customized aroma into your living space to freshen and clean from the ground up (literally). The baking soda helps to absorb unpleasant smells in the carpet, while the essential oils replace the unwanted smell with a naturally pleasant aroma. A variety of essential oils can be used in this recipe. The only caution I would give is to not use sweet orange or tangerine essential oil on light-coloured or white rugs because the orange colour of the essential oil could leave a residue.

METHOD
1. Add the baking soda to a small bowl.
2. Add all the essential oils, then mix with a spoon, trying to break up clumps of essential oils as best as possible.

APPLICATION
1. Using a shaker (you can make one by puncturing small holes in the lid of a mason jar) or a jar, carefully pour the deodorizer over the carpet or rug you want to freshen up.
2. Allow to sit for at least 20 minutes (the longer the better—2 hours is ideal).
3. Vacuum up the deodorizer from the carpet.

STORAGE
Keep extra deodorizer in a covered jar or bowl. Store in a cool, dry place for 2 to 3 months.

Dusting Spray

For when you're going for that "spotless" look (easier said than done).

TIME: 5 minutes

MAKES: 8.45 ounces (250 mL) dusting spray

YOU'LL NEED: a 12-ounce (360 mL) spray bottle

COMPONENTS

1 cup filtered water

2 teaspoons vegetable glycerin

10 drops spruce essential oil

10 drops frankincense essential oil

4 drops lemon essential oil

2 drops lemongrass essential oil

This is an easy multi-purpose spray for dusting and cleaning wood, granite, tile and cement surfaces in the living room. It leaves surfaces looking sophisticated and clean, without using the chemicals found in traditional dusting sprays. The blend I use for this dusting spray is a mix of citrus and woodsy essential oils, which leaves the surfaces of your living room, especially wood surfaces, looking like new.

METHOD

1. Add all components to a spray bottle.

APPLICATION

1. Shake before each use.
2. Spray the surface and wipe immediately afterwards with a soft cloth.

STORAGE

Keep in a cool, dry place away from direct sunlight for up to 2 months.

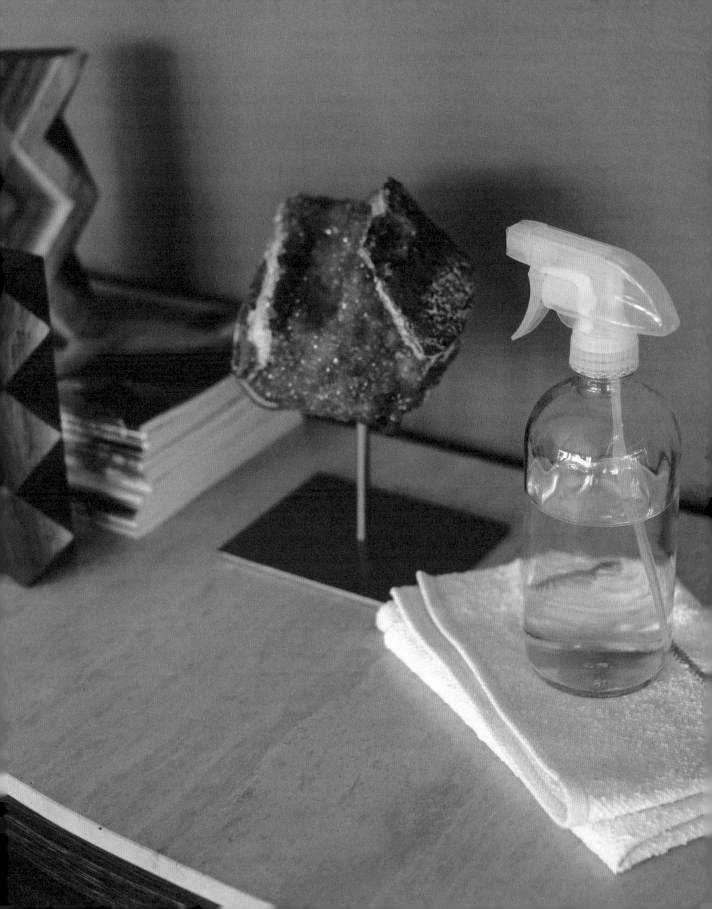

AIR-PURIFYING PLANTS

It's been said that "plant lady" is the new "cat lady." I'm not entirely sure what this means or how I feel about it, but I do know that I have my fair share of plants and that I care about them deeply. Beyond getting us closer to nature and encouraging us to take care of and nurture something, being surrounded by potted plants as often as possible is a great way to keep your air pure. Here are my three favourite plants for keeping the air pure and cleansed in your living and work spaces.

1. RUBBER PLANT
These classy-looking plants are best known for their ability to eliminate carbon monoxide and grow upward, so they'll need space to flourish. They require tons of light, which makes them ideal for sunny apartments and homes with a lot of natural daylight.

2. BAMBOO PALMS
I fell in love with bamboo while in Japan visiting the famous bamboo forest. I would categorize bamboo palms as the most elegant of the air-purifying plants, and these ones are the perfect starter plant—they require only a little care and just a pinch of sunlight. They will eliminate the usual suspects in the air (formaldehyde, benzene and carbon monoxide), and they are totally pet-friendly.

3. ALOE
Having aloe in your home both purifies the air and makes a great addition to DIY beauty products (I've referenced aloe a few times throughout this book). The gel-like substance within the leaves is perfect to soothe a fresh burn or skin irritation. Although they need more light than most plants, they're worth the fuss because they are intense chemical detoxifiers and will start to turn brown when the chemicals in the air have increased, telling you exactly what you need to know.

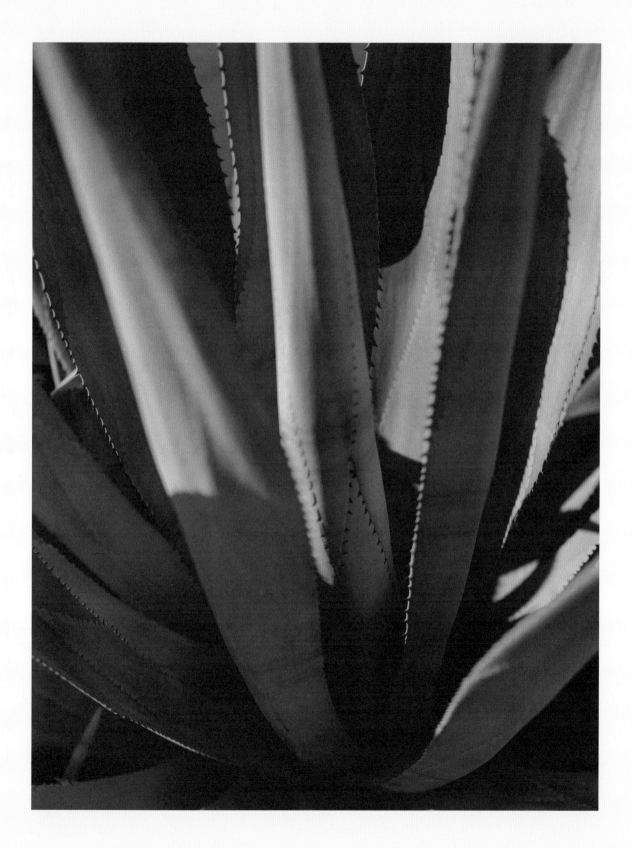

LIVING ROOM DIFFUSER BLENDS

The living room is perhaps the perfect place to showcase your own iconic custom diffuser aromas. I keep a small tray of my favourite essential oils for the living room and blend them together when I get home from work. They're my way of setting the energy in the space and creating a fresh start—it feels great to cleanse the air and my energy after a long day in the office. For the living room, I love using either fresh citrus or herbal essential oils during the day, and more deep and woodsy aromas in the evenings. Using aroma to set a mood and tone is something that has been done for centuries through burning incense or palo santo. Cleansing the air and setting a new intention for the day or evening in ceremony with aroma is a beautiful ritual to incorporate into your living room. I have essential oils I like to diffuse while reading and others I use when I'm cleaning or when people are visiting for wine and dinner. Cueing the brain and body to associate different rituals in the living space with aroma is a powerful way to set the energy for your home.

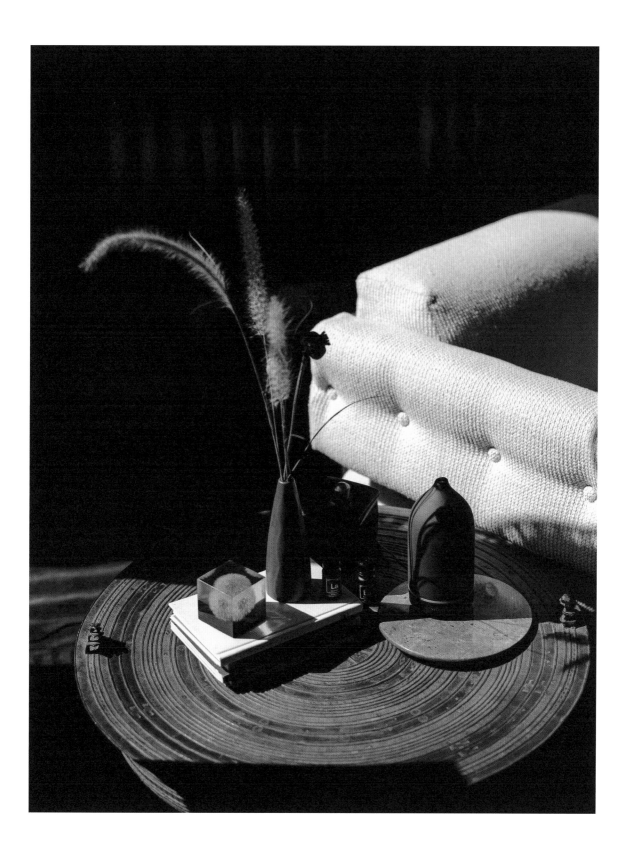

Fresh Start

A blend for when you walk in the door and need to reset your space.

This is a simple blend for when you need to cleanse your space and really make it feel like your own. To reclaim your energy, take a few deep breaths and change your state through scent. Add the components to an ultrasonic diffuser.

10 drops peppermint essential oil

10 drops sweet orange essential oil

Cozy at Home

A blend inspired by the comfort found in a cozy blanket and warm cup of tea (or large glass of red wine).

All that's missing from this blend is your favourite blanket and a good book. I include frankincense because it has been used for centuries as a means of establishing ritual and ceremony. Bergamot provides a cozy and comforting aroma that most people recognize from Earl Grey tea. Lavender provides a beautifully calming aroma that's slightly sedating. Add the components to an ultrasonic diffuser.

9 drops bergamot essential oil

8 drops frankincense essential oil

6 drops lavender essential oil

Cabin Fever in the City

An aroma inspired by the warm and cozy feeling of living the cabin life.

This woodsy blend is perfect for bringing a little nature into your living room. Spruce essential oil has a bright and slightly minty spice to it that I love for bringing the outdoors inside. Pairing it with warmer cedarwood essential oil gives the aroma a full-on cabin vibe. Bergamot essential oil adds a cozy component—the whole blend makes you feel like you just enjoyed some Earl Grey tea after a day of snowshoeing in the Pacific Northwest. Add the components to an ultrasonic diffuser.

8 drops spruce essential oil

6 drops cedarwood essential oil

5 drops bergamot essential oil

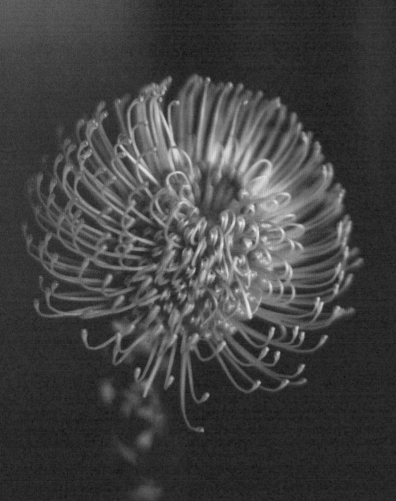

MY DESK ESSENTIALS

I spend an incredible amount of my time at my desk. Building a fast-growing company means that my office feels more like my home, and my workstation has also become quite literally a recharging station. It's a place I've learned to fill with photos, snacks, teas and products that help replenish my energy, both mentally and physically.

GREEN TEA
I find that drinking organic green tea throughout the day gives me more mental clarity and a constant calmer, more focused energy than I get with the quick buzz from coffee. I keep a ceramic jar I purchased in Japan filled with organic green tea bags. I usually have two or three cups of green tea each day and bring it to meetings and planning sessions to keep myself feeling nourished.

EUCALYPTUS AND ROSEMARY ESSENTIAL OILS
The two essential oils I keep on my desk are eucalyptus and rosemary. I've used rosemary essential oil at my desk for years, and it's actually the essential oil that introduced me to the industry. It's been shown to help with memory retention, and I love diffusing it with eucalyptus for a clean, herbal aroma that promotes deep breathing and focus. It makes me feel close to nature and grounded while at my desk.

DARK CHOCOLATE ALMONDS
Dark chocolate–covered almonds have been a part of my life for years. I love the mix of the bitter and the crunch. I keep them in a jar on my desk and have a handful each afternoon around 3 pm with a cup of green tea. This is usually when blood sugar drops and focus lowers for people during the day, so I save easier tasks like emails and phone calls for that time of day—times when I don't need to think as critically.

WATER
The biggest secret in life is water. Drinking more than I think I need has changed my energy, stamina and clarity. Often when we feel a sense of hunger, we're actually thirsty, and by the time we actually feel thirsty, we are dehydrated. I keep a 1-litre glass carafe filled with flavoured water on my desk—usually it holds simply tap water with a sliced lemon or cucumber in it. The flavour makes me drink it more readily. If there is one thing you should keep on your desk, it's water.

REMINDERS

When you're building a project, studying for exams or working at a job, visual reminders that motivate you and remind you of what you are building and why are extremely important. For me, this means a photo of my family and a sticky note that says, "This is not a test." This written reminder means that this life is the real thing—nothing is practice, and the energy, drive, commitment and enthusiasm I have for what I do every day is building the vision, life and legacy that I want to create for myself, our team and my family. These kinds of simple reminders, whatever they might mean to you, are a powerful tool to keep close to you; they will catch your eye and help keep your focus just when you need it.

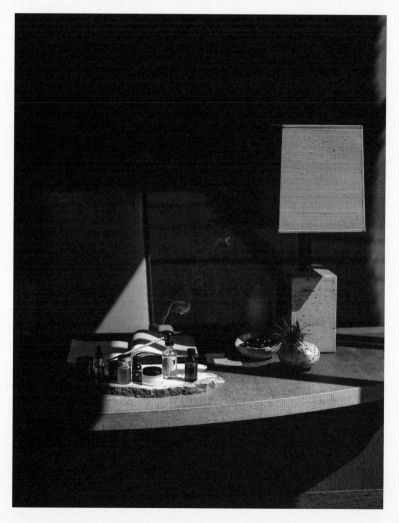

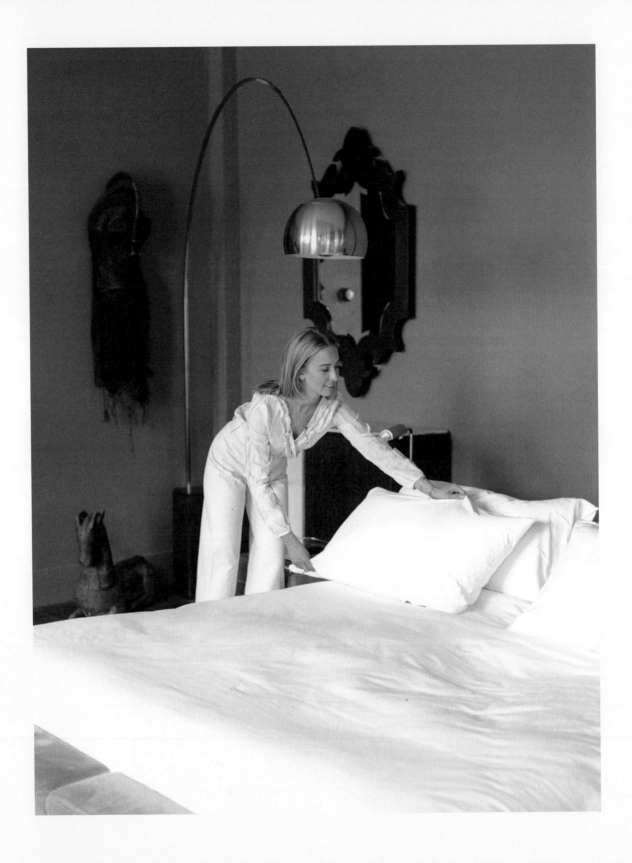

BEDROOM

The bedroom is one of the most common places in the home for people to start experimenting with essential oils. This is because creating a bedtime routine or rituals before you fall asleep is one of the best ways to help get more restorative sleeps and to get the brain and body into the habit of winding down before bed. Essential oils can help create a tone and mood in a room that then cues the brain to start a new practice. Beyond smelling great and creating sleep rituals, using essential oils in the bedroom is extra important because they are completely natural and safe to use on bed sheets and in the laundry. This section shows you ways to incorporate essential oils into your bedroom, laundry and sleep routines.

ESSENTIAL OILS FOR THE BEDROOM

LAVENDER
Possibly the most classic essential oil for the bedroom, lavender has been used as a natural sedative dating back to the 1800s. It's calming and smells like France in a bottle, and I love using it in a diffuser or in homemade sheet sprays for linens and towels. Lavender essential oil also has natural antibacterial and antimicrobial properties, which makes it great for keeping your bedroom clean in the most natural and healthy way.

FRANKINCENSE
Frankincense has been associated with a sense of ceremony and ritual since biblical times, when frankincense and myrrh were left at altars as offerings. This resinous essential oil is great to use when establishing ritual and habits.

YLANG YLANG
This exotic floral essential oil is found in several consistencies—the most precious has a thick, almost sap-like consistency and smells like a million flowers in a bottle. Ylang ylang smells like falling asleep in a hammock underneath a dozen exotic florals on a tropical beach.

LAUNDRY THE NATURAL WAY

Your clothes are on your body at all times. They directly affect your skin, so using natural products to wash, scent and maintain their freshness is important and often overlooked. I like experimenting with essential oils in my laundry routine because they allow me to customize the scent of my clothing while providing a deep, natural clean that's safe on my skin.

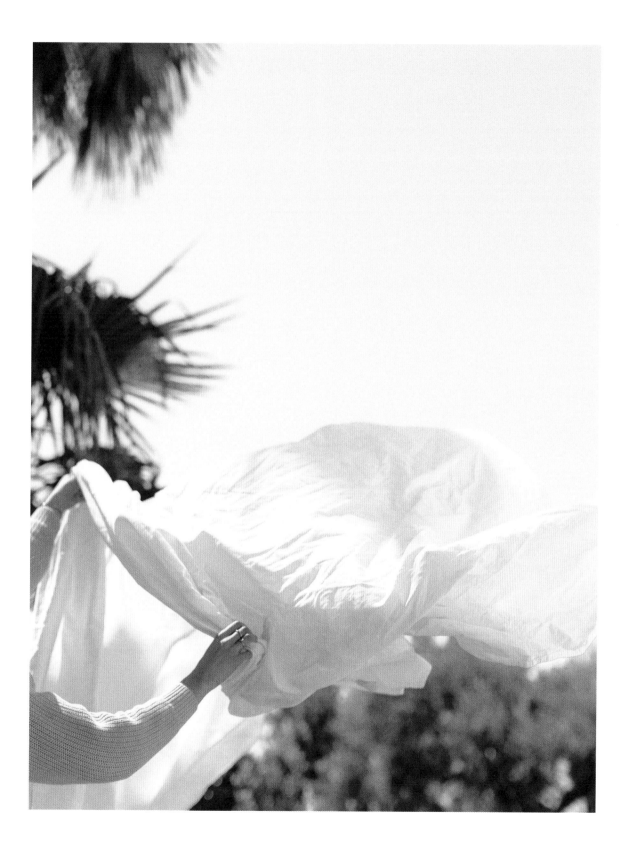

Dryer Sheets

A natural alternative to super-concentrated commercial dryer sheets.

TIME: 10 minutes

MAKES: 5 dryer sheets

YOU'LL NEED: a 16-ounce (480 mL) mason jar or jar with a lid, a spoon and 5 small cloths or fabric scraps

COMPONENTS

1 cup white vinegar

15 drops lavender essential oil

15 drops lemon essential oil

STORAGE

Keep the unused solution in a mason jar covered with a lid away from direct sunlight for up to 2 weeks.

Regular dryer sheets are filled with synthetic aromas and toxins—these chemicals are designed to help keep scents and fragrances on the fabrics. Using homemade dryer sheets lets you use the natural and more interesting aromas of essential oils to create custom scents for your clothing, while feeling a little bit better about what you're putting on your skin.

METHOD

1. Add the vinegar and essential oils to the mason jar and mix with a spoon.

APPLICATION

1. Dip 1 cloth into the mixture in the mason jar. Wring out the cloth to remove excess liquid, then toss it into the dryer with wet clothes. The heat from the dryer will make the vinegar scent go away, and your clothes will be scented with the essential oils.

Dried Lavender Sachets

True self-care is scenting your delicates.

MAKES: 1 sachet

YOU'LL NEED: four 4-inch (10 cm) strips of fabric (cotton, bamboo, linen or silk) or cute socks and string or an elastic band

COMPONENTS

¼ cup dried lavender

5 to 10 drops lavender essential oil

STORAGE

Sachets should stay fresh for up to 6 months.

Keeping your socks and underwear drawer smelling fresh is a little extra that can make the simplest parts of your day (like putting your socks and underwear on) a little more special.

A modern take on scented sheets for your drawers, these lavender sachets are an easy and natural way to add a light scent to your intimates.

METHOD

1. Add the dried lavender to the clean fabric or sock.
2. Sprinkle the lavender essential oil over the dried lavender.
3. Wrap the fabric or sock with string or the elastic band.

APPLICATION

1. Place the sachet in a drawer around socks or underwear.

Linen Spray

Make your pillow the perfect place to lay your head.

TIME: 2 minutes

MAKES: 8.45 ounces (250 mL) linen spray

YOU'LL NEED: a 12-ounce (360 mL) spray bottle

COMPONENTS

1 tablespoon vodka

36 drops lemon essential oil

30 drops spruce essential oil

24 drops lavender essential oil

1 cup filtered water

Linen spray is nice to have around, not only for laundry, but also for bigger items like carpets, bedding, sofas and pillows that can't be run through the washing machine. Even a child's favourite teddy bear needs a little freshening up every once in a while. As a bonus, essential oils don't just mask scent; thanks to their antimicrobial properties, they actually work against the bacteria that cause unpleasant odours. Lavender is a gentle antimicrobial essential oil that's disinfecting and cleansing, while also being calming and uplifting for the mind. Citrus oils like lemon are similar to lavender in their cleansing powers, but they're more invigorating and uplifting. Spruce, a woodsy-smelling oil, is known for its ability to help ground the emotions.

This linen spray is safe for most fabric types, but a small area can be patch tested if there are any concerns. It can be used on bedding, clothing and fabric-covered furniture for a fresh scent.

METHOD

1. Combine the vodka and all the essential oils in the spray bottle and shake to combine.
2. Add the water until the spray bottle is almost full, leaving about ½ inch of space at the top.
3. Cap the bottle and shake again to combine.

APPLICATION

1. Shake well before each use.
2. Liberally spray on fabrics as desired.

STORAGE

Keep in a cool, dry place away from direct sunlight for up to 2 months.

CREATING A BEDROOM OASIS

Your bedroom should be your oasis—it might be filled with kids, laundry, dogs, homework or office notes, but despite the piles of *stuff* taking up space, there are a few simple ways to carve out a little room for yourself. You should set the tone of the room so that it's a space where you refill your body and mind with positivity, rest and relaxation through sleep—or at least so it's a space where you can escape and take a few moments for yourself. Your bedroom should reflect you, and the colours, textures, visual reminders and habits you choose for it should be those that are closest to you.

SHEETS AND PILLOWS

Choosing organic or natural fibre sheets helps you sleep in a healthier way. You spend a good portion of your life in bed—some studies say as much as 50 percent of your life, but for most of us it's at least 30 percent. Linen, hemp or organic cotton sheets help the skin breathe, which is incredibly important while you slumber. Using a natural cleaning agent for your sheets and pillows is also an important practice if you have sensitive skin, as harsh detergents and non-natural fibres can irritate the skin.

ESSENTIAL OILS

I always keep lavender, eucalyptus, frankincense and geranium essential oils beside my bed. They each have different functions, from being used in my diffuser to scenting my sheets and pillow naturally. They are bedside constants, regardless of where I am in the world.

NIGHTSTAND ESSENTIALS

On my nightstand, you'll find lip conditioner, cuticle oil, a tray for my jewellery and a few grounding crystals like smoky quartz and rose quartz.

SALT LAMP AND NATURAL CANDLE

I like having a salt lamp bedside my bed when I'm at home, and if I'm on the road, I'll often bring a small natural travel candle to help make hotel rooms feel more cozy.

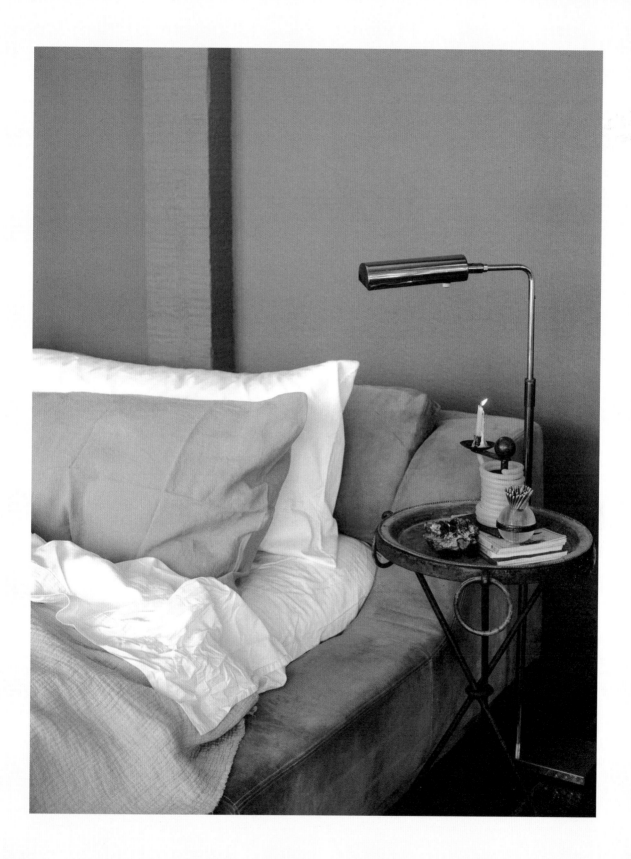

BEDROOM DIFFUSER BLENDS

The bedroom is such a beautiful place in which to create an oasis. Sleep troubles are all too common, and the number of hours of sleep we get each night can become a battle. The amount of sleep we get is often the key factor determining the productivity, perspective and energy we'll have on the following day. These diffuser blends are some of my favourite ways to set the tone for sleep. I put them in the diffuser beside my bed about 1 hour before I plan on going to sleep. Then I close the bedroom door and finish my evening routine—brush my teeth, wash my face and apply my face oils. When I re-enter my bedroom, the scent of the room lets me know it's time for sleep. This diffuser practice has become the focus of my entire evening routine. I hope these blends offer the same results for your evening and usher you into a deep sleep.

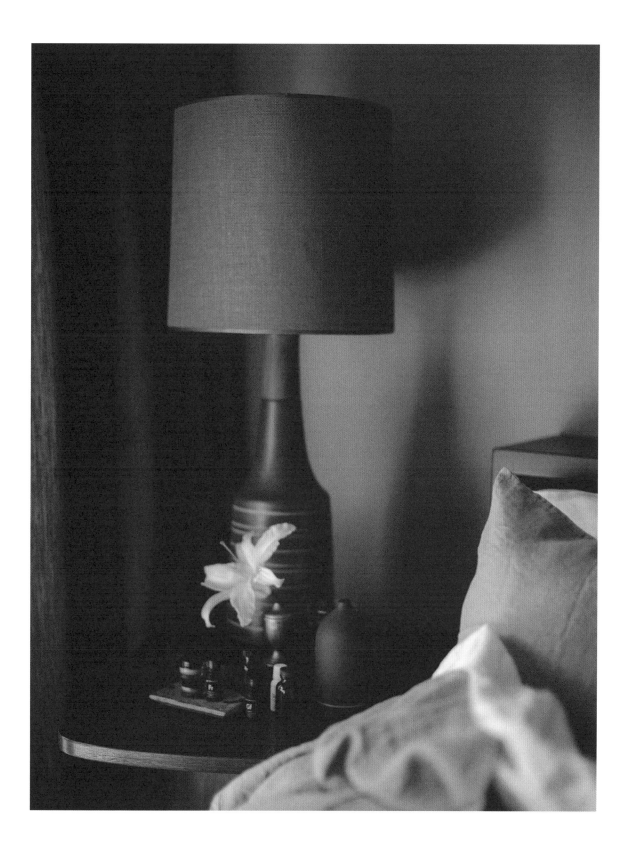

Goddess Time

A blend for when you want to channel your feminine energy.

I wanted to create a blend using the most feminine and powerful essential oils, and what resulted was a gorgeous and well-rounded blend of flowers with woodsy herbal aroma. I suggest using this blend in the evening to help calm and ground yourself, while journaling or in the morning as you get ready so you can start your day in a positive and feminine mindset. Geranium is a very feminine aroma that gives beautiful depth and cleanliness to the blend, making it grounding yet also uplifting. Lavender essential oil is a favourite for any blend that may be used during reflection. Ylang ylang is one of the most feminine of the floral essential oils; it has a powdery floral aroma and a slightly thicker consistency. Cedarwood essential oil helps provide a level of clear thinking and grounded energy inspired by its rooted status in nature. Frankincense is our ceremonial essential oil—I like to use it while journaling or setting intentions. It's associated with the root chakra (in Ayurvedic medicine), and its aroma can inspire energy and strength from a grounded place. Add the components to an ultrasonic diffuser.

7 drops geranium essential oil

6 drops lavender essential oil

2 drops ylang ylang essential oil

2 drops frankincense essential oil

1 drop cedarwood essential oil

Beauty Sleep

A blend that's as gorgeous as you are.

While I love putting on my diffuser an hour or so before bedtime, I also love running it through the night while I sleep. In the Beauty section of this book, I shared many ways you can benefit from the properties of essential oils by adding them to your skincare regimen. I like to think of this blend as the non-topical version of that—scenting the air with some of my favourite essential oils for beauty gives *beauty sleep* a whole new meaning. This is a soft and sensual blend that can help lull you to sleep while beautifying the air around you. Add the components to an ultrasonic diffuser.

6 drops geranium essential oil

5 drops cedarwood essential oil

2 drops frankincense essential oil

Sweet Dreams, Darling

A blend that helps you drift into dreamland.

This diffuser blend was created by my mom and dad (the true test kitchen and critics of all our products). After years of experimenting with oils, this has become their go-to in the evening to get a restful sleep. When I visit our family home on Vancouver Island, the house usually starts to smell like this blend around 10 pm, and I know that Mom has put on her diffuser in preparation for bedtime. I had to share our family bedside diffuser blend, as it's an incredibly powerful scent memory for me—plus, it smells heavenly and immediately puts me in the mood to wind down. Add the components to an ultrasonic diffuser.

6 drops lavender essential oil

5 drops cedarwood essential oil

2 drops frankincense essential oil

1 drop lemongrass essential oil

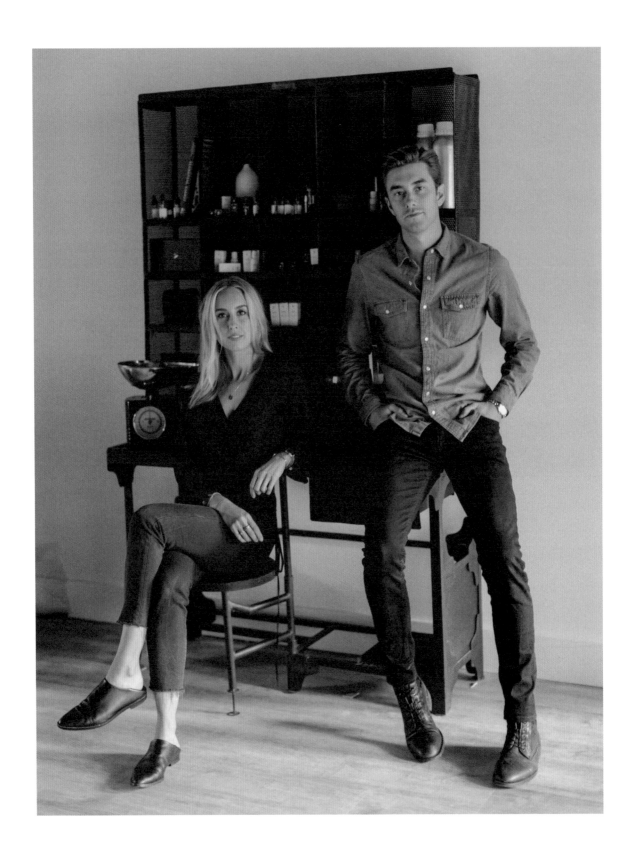

ACKNOWLEDGEMENTS

This book was built by a group of incredibly talented individuals . . .

The first I want to thank is Alex Falconer, whose talent for words as well as bright spirit, creativity, and skillfully diligent and brilliant mind helped craft and edit the tone and flow of this book.

Thank you to Britney Gill for capturing the process through photographs in a way that only she can. She is gifted and talented beyond measure.

Thank you to Jasmien Hamed for her styling and for understanding and living fully the concept of the world we aim to create for women—and for doing it all with so much ease.

Thank you to Jenna Vaandering for her incredible illustrative talent and for truly shaping the vitruvi aesthetic.

Thank you to Lori and Jim for being the most gracious hosts.

Thank you to my brother, Sean, for being the best teammate and cofounder. Nothing would exist without his vision, drive, intuition, skill and ability to learn faster than anyone I've ever met. It is truly an honour to work with him.

And thank you to the vitruvi team for their endless focus, dedication and compassion for our customers and products. These pages were inspired by what they have built and the lighthearted spirit they have brought to the process.

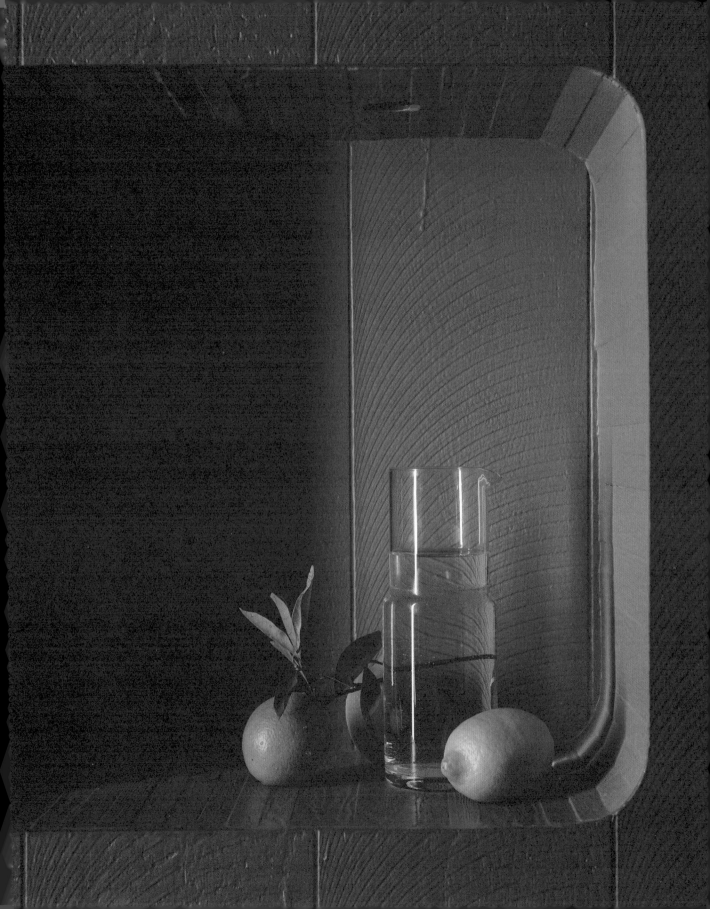

INDEX